the Baby Bistro

Child-Approved Recipes and Expert Nutrition Advice for the First Year

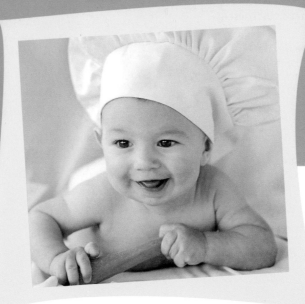

Christina Schmidt, M.S. Nutrition

Bull Publishing Company
Boulder, Colorado

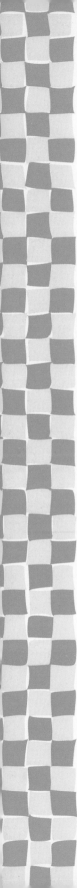

Bull Publishing Company

P.O. Box 1377
Boulder, CO 80306
(800) 676-2855
www.bullpub.com

Book design and production by Shannon Bodie, Lightbourne, Inc.

Design concept by John Betlejewski

Illustrations by Steve Veach

Photography by Peter McQuarry, McQuarry Photography (except where noted)

Printed in Canada by Friesens

Distributed to the Trade by
Independent Publishers Group
814 North Franklin Street
Chicago, IL 60610

Library of Congress Cataloging-in-Publication Data

Schmidt, Christina, 1970–
The baby bistro : child-approved recipes and expert nutrition advice for the first year /
by Christina Schmidt.
        p. cm.
Includes index.
        ISBN 978-1-933503-18-9
   1. Infants--Nutrition.   2. Cookery (Baby foods) I. Title.
RJ216.S398 2009
641.5'6222--dc22

2008048948

The trademarks referenced within this body of work are the property of their respective owners, are not affiliated with this author, and are mentioned merely as suggested food item options for the reader.

The suggested brands and food items mentioned within this body of work are for illustrative purposes only, and the author does not warrant their fitness to the reader or others. It is always wise to check with your health care provider with respect to fitness, ingredients, and potential allergic reactions to certain food groups or combinations.

Acknowledgments a la Mode

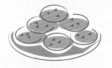

My loving family—Grandma B., mom Susan, sister Gretchen, brother Pete, and husband Neil

My little tasters—Adam, Grant, Evan, Trent, and, of course, my dog Cedar

My forever friends—Neil, Robyn, Karol, Mary, Anne, Erika, Kalai, and Luisa

My genius designer—John Betlejewski, Design Touch

My imaginative illustrator—Steve Veach, Veach Illustration and Design

My gifted and patient photographer—Peter McQuarry, McQuarry Photography

My brilliant reviewers—Iris Castañeda-Van Wyk, M.D., Daniel Brennan, M.D., Myron I. Liebhaber, M.D., Erika Conner, R.D., Patti Stoffers, C.N.P., Robyn Shields, D.D.S.

My publishing dream team—Jim, Betsy, George, Shannon, and Dianne

The Menu

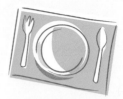

Chef – Christina E. Schmidt, M.S., N.E.

Acknowledgments a la Mode iii
My journey from carrots to a calling vii

Starters ... *Pre-birth pointers for moms-to-be* 1

Recommended weight gain during pregnancy 2
Nutrient needs for moms 2
Popular diets—hopeless or healthy? 5
Nutrient no-no's for moms 6

First Course ... *Preparing for feeding baby: health and safety* 9

Allergy advice 10
Beverage beware 12
Bottle boundaries 14
Chancy cheeses 14
Can the cocoa 15
Choking checks 15
Egg education 16
Fishy fish 17
Foolish fats 20
Funky fruits 21
Hold the honey . . . and the corn syrup 22
Meat monsters 22
Nut notes 24
Opt for organic 24
Plastic priorities 27
Skip the salt, sugar and spices 28
Vexing veggies 29
Watch the wheat 30
Shopping smarts 31

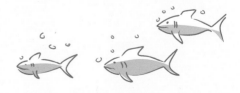

Entrées . . . **Birth to four months**   **35**

    Nutrient needs   36
    Breast milk   36
    Medications and breast-feeding   41
    Formula fundamentals...Menu choices   43

Entrées . . . **Four to six months**   **47**

    Nutrient needs   48
    Signals for solids   49
    Serving suggestions for solids   50
    Solids du Jour   51
    Solids from scratch...Try your hand at homemade purées   52
    Bistro recipes...Purées   54

Entrées . . . **Six to eight months**   **61**

    Nutrient needs   62
    Serving suggestions   63
    More on the menu   65

Entrées . . . **Eight to twelve months**   **83**

    Nutrient needs   84
    Serving suggestions   84
    More on the menu   85

Á la Carte . . . **Supplements**   **103**

    For the baby   104
    For the vegan baby   109
    For pregnant and breast-feeding moms   110
    For pregnant and breast-feeding vegan moms   116
    Supplement savvy   117

Desserts . . . **Savor the sweetness**   **121**

    Appendices
       1. A Spoonful of sources   123
       2. Shopping simplicity   125
       3. A blend of measurements   129

    Index
       Subject index   130
       Recipe index   134

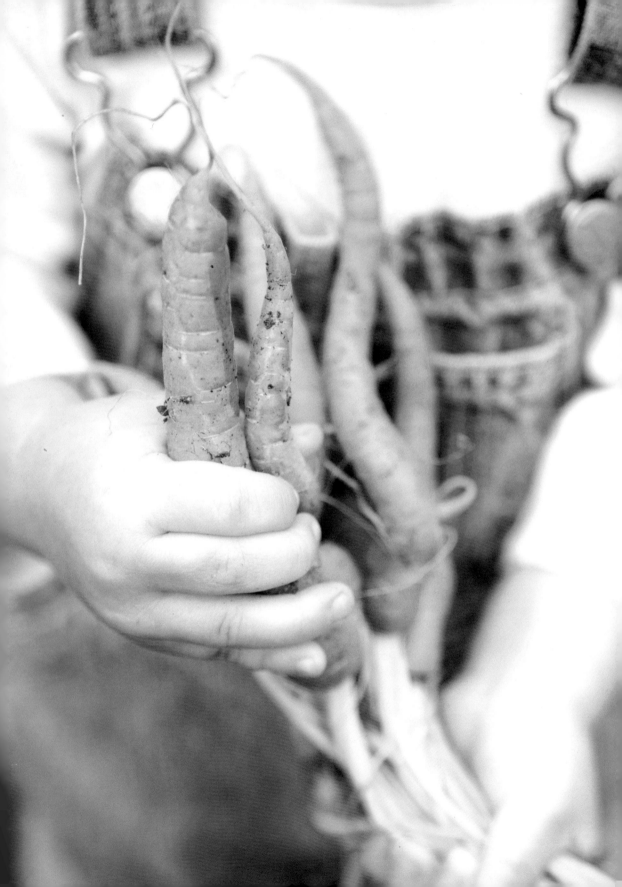

My Journey

From carrots to a calling

If you are pregnant or have a newborn, you are probably overwhelmed with thousands of questions about raising babies. Which car seat is best? Is there a right way to change a diaper? How do you know if your baby is hungry or just fussy? Instinct, childhood experience, trial and error, friends, and expert advice may be some of your resources in discovering the answers.

One thing I have realized in life is that it is impossible to know everything. Right now, with a new baby to nurture, you may be feeling more humble than ever in your realm of expertise!

My Journey

I chose to learn a lot about something that has always fascinated me—nutrition. My childhood memories involve planting seeds, tending gardens, and eating fresh fruits and vegetables, with my mother in the background explaining the important vitamins in each. "Carrots help build strong eyesight," she repeated almost daily.

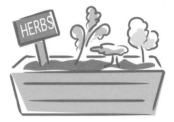

In school, I set out to decipher nutritional facts from fiction. I studied alternative nutrition science, earning a Nutrition Educator certification, and from there I moved into mainstream nutrition and food science, gaining a Master of Science degree. In my graduate work, I discovered that my passion resided in the interplay of nutrients and crucial developmental stages of life.

Shortly after graduation, my friends and my sister began having babies and asking me questions about what, how, and when to feed their newborns. I became concerned with the gap between the findings in nutrient research that had existed for years and the awareness among parents outside the academic environment. I searched bookstores for a complete, easy to comprehend, fun infant feeding book to suggest to my pregnant friends, but could find nothing.

My sister and I were taking her seven-month-old, Adam, for a walk along Shoreline Park one sunny day and talking about how moms were hungry for credible infant nutritional information. My first product, the Baby Bistro Box®, was born from that discussion. The "box" contained infant feeding advice written in a recipe-like format on cards. The Toddler Bistro Box® followed two years later, as my mommy readers asked what to do after year one!

The Baby Bistro and *Toddler Bistro* books represent my passion and commitment to put important information about feeding infants and toddlers into the hands of parents and caregivers. Of course, you cannot be the perfect parent and know everything, but hopefully these books will empower you with the knowledge you'll need to build a healthful foundation for your growing family that lasts a lifetime.

The Baby Bistro menu is your gourmet tour to healthy feeding. Starters and First Course prepare you with important nutritional and safety information as you dive into the Entrées section, where you'll progress through your baby's feeding stages and try some babylicious recipes. Á la Carte suggests side portions of information about supplements and nutrients to enhance the feeding experience for you and your baby. Desserts are just that—the final course that is a surprise that you'll have to wait for until you finish your "meal." Don't even think about cheating and reading the end first! All in all, this Baby Bistro is about helping you successfully run your own exclusive bistro for your baby. *Happy feeding!*

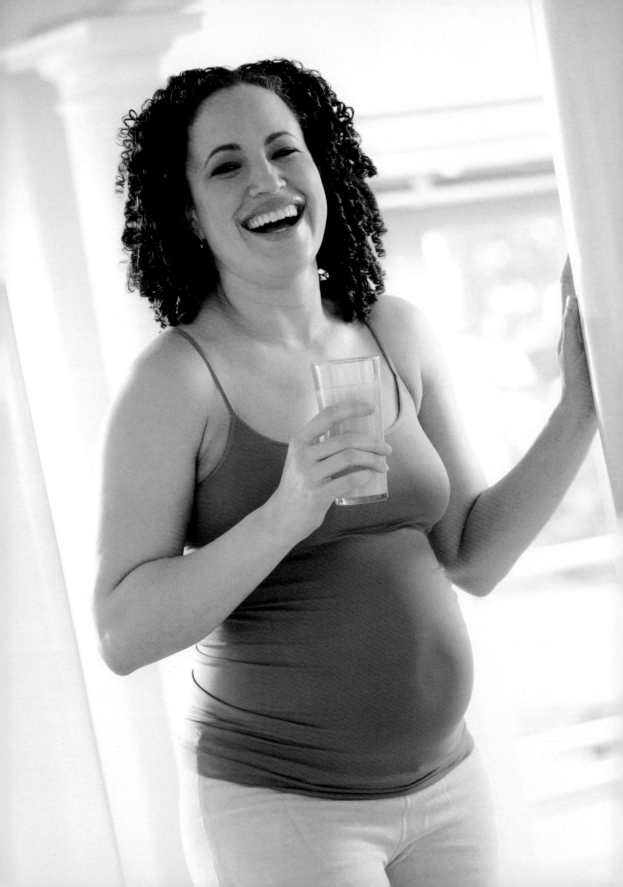

Starters

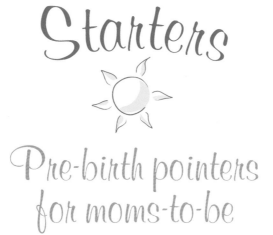

Pre-birth pointers for moms-to-be

Preparing for your baby's arrival while you are pregnant means trying to be as organized as possible before your life happily turns upside down, sleep deprivation strikes, and time to read and remember things escapes your daily reality. The Starters are first on the bistro menu, with recommendations for weight gain during pregnancy and nutrition tips to help you to navigate your way through your pregnancy diet confidently.

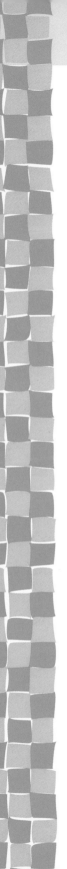

Starters

Recommended weight gain during pregnancy

According to recommendations from The American College of Obstetricians and Gynecologists Institute of Medicine, women with normal weight should gain twenty-five to thirty-five pounds (11.5 to 16.0 kg) in pregnancy; those who are underweight, twenty-eight to forty pounds (12.5 to 18.0 kg); and overweight women should gain fifteen to twenty-five pounds (7.0 to 11.5 kg). Most of your weight gain should occur during your second and third trimesters. Your doctor can help monitor your progress as well as counsel you if you have special needs or are pregnant with multiples. In general, ditch that latest diet and just concentrate on eating healthy, nutritious foods!

The objective is to maximize your nutrients per calorie, regardless of whether you are having trouble keeping foods down or are ravenous.

Nutrient needs for moms

During pregnancy and breast-feeding, your body requires a boost in protein and energy to support your growing baby and to keep all of your systems on GO as well! Proteins are paramount in building nearly everything necessary for human growth, such as muscles, skin, organs, bones, and the immune and nervous systems. You should aim for a protein intake range of sixty to seventy grams per day.

Add an extra nutritious snack into your daily diet as well. You need to take in a few more calories than prior to your pregnancy to support additional energy requirements, especially during the second and third trimesters and during breast-feeding.

	Protein	Calories
Pregnant	71 grams/day	+300/day
Lactating birth to 12 months	71 grams/day	+500/day

Pack in the protein

Make sure you've added plenty of meats, poultry, fish, dairy products, soy products, beans, eggs, whole grains, and nuts to your diet. Use this list of protein-rich foods to guide you in your choices:

4 ounces chicken = 34 grams

4 ounces fish = 30 grams

4 ounces hamburger = 28 grams

1 cup tofu = 18 grams

1 cup kidney beans = 16 grams

1 cup fruit yogurt = 10 grams

1/2 cup edamame = 10 grams

2 tablespoons peanut butter = 9 grams

1 cup skim milk = 8 grams

1 ounce cheese = 7 grams

1 large egg = 6 grams

1 cup white rice = 6 grams

1 cup broccoli = 3 grams

Factor in fabulous fiber foods

Everyone should include fiber in their diet. Fiber protects against certain cancers, helps control cholesterol ratios, evens out blood sugar levels, combats weight gain, and allows the digestive system to function smoothly. Pregnant women may be more prone to the lovely discomforts of constipation and hemorrhoids. Eating high-fiber foods daily will help to keep your digestion on a regular track. Aim for about 28 grams per day. Natural sources of fiber are fruits, vegetables, beans, and whole grains.

Not all fats are the enemy

Healthy fats are available in a variety of delicious foods and are an important part of your diet. Fat stores energy, transports vitamins, supports healthy skin, and is vital to the brain, the central nervous system and your visual development. The skinny on fat is to allow saturated fats (found mostly in meat, whole-fat dairy, egg yolks, and palm and coconut oils) to be only a very small portion of your diet. Instead, favor unsaturated fats. These include monounsaturated fats and polyunsaturated fats, especially the two "essential" fats, which are fats our bodies cannot make.

Foods like avocados, peanut butter, and olive and canola oils are high in monounsaturated fats. The essential fats are linoleic (omega-6) fats and linolenic (omega-3) fats. Try to include about 13 grams per day of omega-6 fats and 1.4 grams per day of omega-3 fats in your diet during pregnancy. The omega-6 fats are found mostly in nuts, seeds, and vegetable and seed oils. The omega-3 fats are found in soybeans, flaxseeds, walnuts, wheat germ, and cold-water fish. The main omega-3 in cold-water fish is DHA, which is vital for your baby's brain and retinal development. Pregnant and breast-feeding moms, babies, and young children should exclude certain fish from their seafood selections (see First Course, Fishy Fish, p. 17, for a full listing).

Avoid partially hydrogenated fats (transfats). These fats may interfere with your baby's normal course of growth and nervous system development (see First Course, Foolish Fats, p. 20).

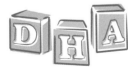 Don't forget to take your prenatal vitamin and DHA supplement! (See Á la Carte, p. 105.)

Popular diets—hopeless or healthy?

If you follow a specific diet, you may be wondering if it is safe to continue throughout your pregnancy.

Vegan or vegetarian diets

Vegan and vegetarian diets are healthy diets that offer plenty of nutrition for the healthy birth of your baby. Vegan diets exclude all meats, fish, dairy, and eggs. Vegan moms should pay extra attention to include enough protein, zinc, iron, calcium, and vitamins D and B12, because these nutrients are primarily in animal-based foods.

Vegetarians usually eat some foods from the animal kingdom such as dairy, fish, or eggs. If you do not eat fish, your body may have suboptimal levels of DHA, and you should take a supplement. Fruits and veggies naturally offer some calcium and iron. Many vegan foods and beverages are fortified with vitamin B12, zinc, calcium, and vitamin D. Your prenatal vitamin and DHA supplement are good insurance policies to cover dietary nutrient gaps.

Macrobiotic diets

If you practice this diet and plan to raise your baby on it, please think again! Macrobiotic diets are very restrictive and are not recommended for pregnant women or infants because they do not contain proper levels of energy, nutrients, vitamins, and minerals essential for normal growth and development. Nutrients lacking in this diet include protein, vitamin B12, iron, and calcium. Babies on this diet are at risk for rickets and failure to thrive.

Low carbohydrate, fruitarian, or other fad diet regimens

These diets are nutritionally inadequate and do not support the needs of a growing baby or pregnant mom. If you must experiment with them, wait until after pregnancy and breast-feeding. Pregnancy is your best excuse to put off dieting!

Nutrient no-no's for moms

Certain foods may harbor bacteria, parasites, or viruses that may put your health and the health of your baby at risk. Here is the story behind why you have to skip some of your favorite food indulgences!

Listeria monocytogenes, Salmonella, and *Toxoplasma gondii* are bacteria that may cause illnesses such as listeriosis, salmonella poisoning, or toxoplasmosis. Pregnant women, their unborn babies, and newborns are at an increased risk of becoming infected. Infection may develop into serious health risks during pregnancy and after the birth of your baby.

Avoid ready-to-eat foods such as deli-style lunch meats and poultry, refrigerated meat spreads, refrigerated smoked seafood, bologna, hot dogs, fermented and dry sausage, deli salads and spreads, and pâtés. Also avoid raw or undercooked meat, poultry, seafood, raw eggs, raw homemade cookie dough, unpasteurized milk or juice, and soft cheeses like Brie, blue-veined, feta, Camembert, Roquefort, or Mexican soft cheeses (queso blanco, queso fresco, queso de crea, panela, asadero).

Shelf-stable or canned pâté and smoked seafood and pasteurized soft cheeses like cream cheese, ricotta, and cottage cheese are fine to eat. Yes, you still get to have your bagel with schmear, just no lox!

Skip the raw sushi, raw shellfish, and sashimi, and retreat from raw meat such as in those delicious appetizers like tartars or carpaccios. In addition to the bacteria previously mentioned, raw fish may contain the hepatitis A virus as well as parasites that are dangerous to you and your baby. Sushi prepared with cooked fish is OK.

Go for sproutless sandwiches and wraps. Despite their health benefits, alfalfa, clover, and radish sprouts unfortunately may carry *Salmonella, E. coli*, and the canavanine toxin.

Adopting smart kitchen habits also helps to keep your foods bug-free. Set your refrigerator temperature to 40°F (4°C) and reheat meats to steaming hot. Refrigerate foods that may spoil within two hours after they have been prepared or eaten. Wash your hands before preparing food and keep pets away from culinary surfaces. Check www.fsis.usda.gov for more information.

One more thing you can check off your to-do list while you are pregnant is your call to the local public works or water board to inquire about the fluoride content in your tap water, or check My Water's Fluoride at http://apps.nccd.cdc.gov/MWF/Index.asp. Adequate levels of fluoride in your local water are between 0.7 to 1.2 parts per million (ppm). If levels are lower than 0.3 ppm, and you plan to use tap water for formula or to drink when breast-feeding, you may need to give your baby a fluoride supplement at six months. Consult with your pediatrician or a pediatric dentist. Fluoride is essential in building strong teeth and bones (see Á la Carte, p. 108).

If you tap into a well for your water, verify that it contains less than 10 ppm of nitrate/nitrogen. Higher levels of nitrates in water used for baby formula or for cooking baby foods may interfere with the oxygen supply to your baby's body tissues (see Vexing Veggies, p. 29).

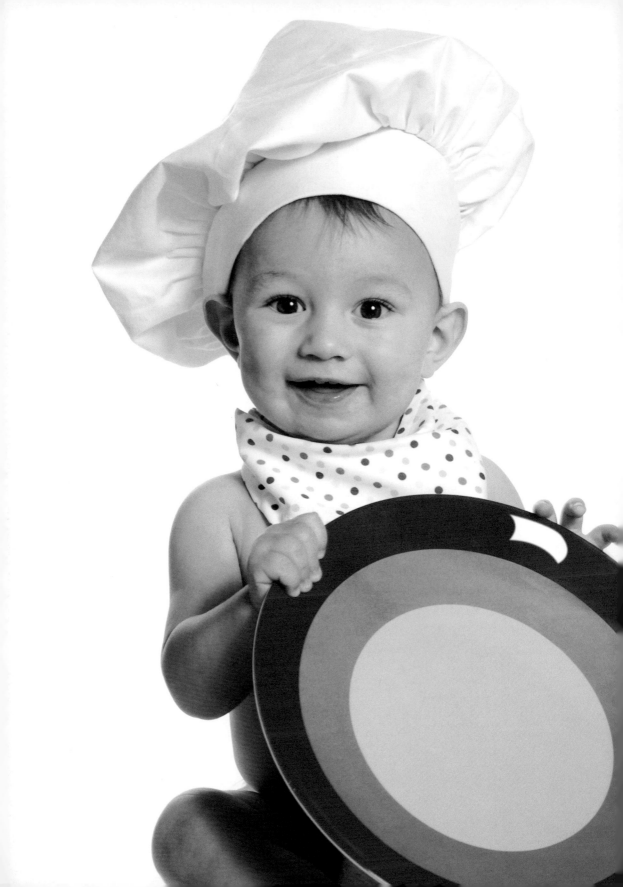

First Course

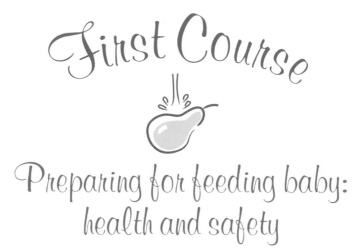

Preparing for feeding baby: health and safety

Is organic food really better? Can I give my baby carton-brand cow milk? Which fish are healthy and safe for babies? What is the real deal with trans-fats? As a new parent or a grandparent (a.k.a. free babysitter), you crave information about how to protect and raise a healthy baby. Many of my readers have said they never really understood certain nutrition topics such as food allergies, trans-fats, or high-mercury fish until they had gone through this "First Course."

The Baby Bistro First Course serves up some food-safety specifics to expand your knowledge palate and launch you confidently into feeding your baby and selecting food.

Allergy advice

For the experts who research childhood allergies and methods to prevent, delay, or treat symptoms, the jury is still out on the best approach. Current scientific consensus is that WHEN parents introduce common allergenic foods to their babies has no impact on whether or not their child develops allergies. Evidence indicates that for high-risk children who have a sibling or parent with allergies, waiting to offer certain foods for the first year or more may delay, but not prevent, allergy onset. Basically, we cannot trick our genes, but we may be able to downplay them a bit.

If your baby displays hypersensitivity such as dermatitis during the first four months of age before you introduce solid foods, ask your pediatrician about holding off on offering the common food allergens.

Food allergies in most children resolve by five or six years of age; however, allergies to peanuts, nuts, and seafood may last a lifetime.

The Bistro Big Eight allergenic foods

Proteins in foods may provoke an immune reaction known as a food allergy. If your baby develops a reaction after eating solids or nursing, certain foods are most likely to be the cause. It helps to know the lineup of the most common food allergens when you and your doctor are tracking the root of a mystery rash or wheezing. Introducing the Big Eight:

- Eggs
- Tree nuts
- Soy
- Milk

- Fish
- Wheat
- Peanuts
- Shellfish

Other foods that are known to trigger allergic reactions are berries, especially strawberries, citrus, tomatoes, corn, kiwi, sesame, and mustard seed.

Symptoms

Allergic symptoms may occur within a few minutes to hours of eating, usually after two or three exposures to the food. Common symptoms are hives, rash, itching, eczema, facial swelling, wheezing, nasal congestion, coughing, asthma, diarrhea, vomiting, and stomach pain. Hives are the most common allergic reaction.

If you suspect a food allergy, eliminate the food(s) and contact your health care provider. Your baby may need to be tested for allergies.

Tips for allergy-prone babies

Does your baby have a parent or sibling with allergies (food, environmental, asthma, or eczema)? Approximately 80 percent of allergy-prone children are allergic to one or two foods. If you have an allergy-prone baby, read on for some hints that may help improve some allergic symptoms!

Eating a diet rich in zinc, vitamin D, vitamin E, antioxidants, and omega 3 fats found in low-mercury fish during pregnancy and breast-feeding may help to reduce potential wheezing in your baby's toddler years.

If, after nursing, you suspect that your baby has symptoms of an allergic reaction, talk to your pediatrician about excluding allergenic foods from your diet. Research indicates that this may improve symptoms of colic during a baby's first six weeks of life.

Breast-feeding exclusively for at least the first four months appears to protect high-risk infants from developing more severe allergies and asthma.

If you are not able to nurse, feeding your baby an extensively hydrolyzed formula instead of regular cow or soy protein formulas may be beneficial to prevent or delay allergic skin reactions.

Check www.foodallergy.org for more information.

Beverage beware

Your baby's beverage menu during the first year is fairly exclusive. Breast milk and baby formula should be the primary picks and the following liquids are best left off the list.

Commercial cow's milk (carton brands)

No servings: birth to twelve months
The protein in cow's milk, called casein, is an allergen. Cow's milk

delivers overabundant amounts of protein, salt, potassium, and chloride, putting too much stress on your baby's immature kidneys. Cow's milk does not provide adequate levels of absorbable iron, zinc, essential fatty acids, vitamin E, and vitamin C for normal growth and development. Cow's milk is best for baby cows!

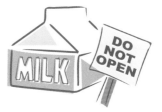

Commercial soy milk

No servings: birth to twelve months
Like cow's milk, soy milk delivers too much protein and salt, overworking baby kidneys. Soy milk also does not provide the necessary levels of absorbable zinc and iron to grow healthy babies.

Using these milks as ingredients in recipes for nonallergic babies is fine!

Other "milks"

No servings: birth to twelve months
These include goat milk and milk imposters such as from rice, nuts, seeds, nondairy creamers, and water-based cereal porridge. These milks do not contain adequate amounts of calories, protein, vitamins, and minerals to support growth. If you are nursing and prefer to drink these milks, make sure that you choose brands fortified with calcium, vitamin D, folic acid, and vitamin B12 in order to provide adequate nutrients for you and your baby during breast-feeding.

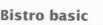

Bistro basic

Breast milk is best.
Don't mess with the milks!

Fruit juice

No servings: birth to twenty-four months
Fruit juice flunks out of the Baby Bistro diet! Full of
sugar, it causes diarrhea and dental decay, encourages
a preference for sweet beverages, and increases risk for
obesity. Fruit juice sacrifices nutrients for sugar and has
been associated with failure to thrive in infants who drink
large quantities. If you choose to offer juice, use only unsweetened
juices, and because of possible allergies, do not offer citrus juices for
the first twelve months. Dilute all juices with water and serve them
in a cup, not a bottle, to prevent tooth decay. Limit serving sizes to a
1/2 cup (4 ounces or 120 milliliters) of diluted juice per day.

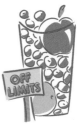

Bottle boundaries

Do not allow your baby to fall asleep with a bottle or have
unlimited access to a bottle or sippy cup. Constant sucking
may affect palate formation and speech, and overexposure to the
sugar in milk can cause tooth decay. Your goal should be no bottle
after twelve months.

If you are nursing and intend to bottle-feed during the first year to
meet the demands of work and life, introduce the bottle early so that
your baby does not become a breast snob!

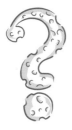

Chancy cheeses

Soft, unpasteurized cheeses are a no-no! Fabulous,
gourmet cheeses such as Brie, feta, blue-veined,

Roquefort, Camembert, Mexican-style (queso blanco, queso fresco, queso de crea, panela, asadero), and goat cheese may contain *listeria* bacteria, a Baby Bistro reject! Soft cheeses with a pasteurized label such as cream cheese or ricotta cheese are safe for your baby cheese-o-philes.

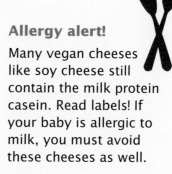

Allergy alert!

Many vegan cheeses like soy cheese still contain the milk protein casein. Read labels! If your baby is allergic to milk, you must avoid these cheeses as well.

Can the cocoa

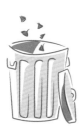

Avoid feeding your baby chocolate or any cocoa product for the first twelve months. Chocolate is an allergen and contains caffeine. If you are nursing, you may indulge in your occasional chocolate fix, but babies will not miss it during year one until they smear that first chocolate cake all over their faces.

Choking checks

Be careful with vegetable and fruit skins, raw vegetables, whole grapes, dried fruits, raisins, popcorn, hot dog slices, snack chips, whole beans, nuts, stringy meats, chunks of meats and cheeses, pickles, and BIG BITES!

Foods such as these that are chunky and hard to chew are beyond babies' swallowing expertise and may cause choking!

15

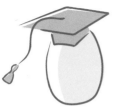

Egg education

Eggs are a rich source of nutrients but may be problematic for some babies. Exercise your new egg knowledge when serving up this dish.

Egg whites

No servings: birth to eight months

Eggs store most of their protein, albumin, in the white. Albumin is allergenic. Babies without a family history of allergy may enjoy a tasty egg scramble when you introduce other meats and proteins at seven to eight months.

Egg yolks

No servings: birth to six months

The yolk is allergenic, but less so than the white. You may include cooked yolks on the menu when you introduce other regular solid foods to your baby at around six months.

Allergy alert!

If your baby has a strong family history of allergies, or has already shown sensitivity reactions such as eczema during the first few months, wait or use caution in serving eggs during the first two years. Egg substitutes still contain egg protein and should be avoided as well.

Chef's secret

Egg substitute in recipes: Mix 1 1/2 tablespoons water with 1 1/2 tablespoons oil and 1 1/2 teaspoon baking powder.

Fishy fish

Overall, fish have many healthy benefits, but keep these following factors in mind when selecting seafood for babies.

Check fish advisories before serving recreationally caught fish from lakes, rivers, or the ocean. Even though Uncle Bob says it's the best, his prized fresh catch that he proudly presents from his annual fishing expedition may not be safe for babies.

Check www.edf.org and www.epa.gov/waterscience/fish for a listing of fish advisories. Look for "Seafood Safe" labels in supermarkets and restaurants.

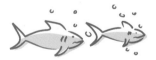

Bistro basic

Best choice for tuna? Use canned, chunk-light skipjack tuna. Canned, white albacore tuna contains higher levels of mercury. The Federal Drug Administration (FDA) and Environmental Protection Agency (EPA) advise women who are pregnant, nursing, or may become pregnant, and children under twelve, that they may eat up to twelve ounces of low-mercury fish per week. They allow six of those ounces to be from albacore tuna. Due to conflicting research on mercury levels in canned tuna, however, it may be prudent to completely avoid this selection. Try substituting canned wild salmon for a similar tasting, yet safer dish.

Bistro Bests **Try these fish:** Pacific sole, salmon (see Scoop on Salmon, p. 19), U.S. tilapia, catfish, turbot, herring, mahi-mahi, sardines, red snapper, rainbow trout, flounder, farmed striped bass, pollock, Pacific halibut, and sablefish

Avoid swordfish, shark, tuna (including ahi steaks), gold or white snapper, king mackerel, marlin, bluefish, wild striped bass, walleye, and tilefish.

No servings: birth to twenty-four months
These predator fish can store dangerous levels of mercury. The older, larger fish contain the highest amounts. Mercury poisoning in humans causes potential heart damage, delayed development, nerve disorders, and mental retardation. The first two years of life are crucial for brain development.

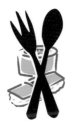

Raw fish

No servings: birth to twenty-four months
Sorry, no sushi! Raw fish can carry the hepatitis virus, bacteria and parasites, invaders that your baby's immune system is not ready to battle.

Shellfish

No servings: birth to twenty-four months
Shrimp, crab, lobster, mussels, clams, crayfish, etc. are common allergens. Although babies with no family history of allergy are at little risk of being allergic to shellfish, many equally healthy fish options are less allergenic.

Allergy alert!
If your family has a strong history of allergy, or if your baby has already exhibited allergic sensitivities, avoid or use caution in serving fish and shellfish for the first three years.

The scoop on salmon

Farmed salmon
No servings: birth to two years

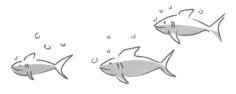

Wild salmon
Start servings: eight months

To farm or not to farm? Good question! Being at the top of the food chain, we care that our favorite fish eat healthy foods. Wild salmon feast on deep ocean krill, green algae, and other small fish. Farmed salmon eat concentrated fish meal and fish oil. Salmon feed is harvested from waters close to shore areas that are potentially contaminated with carcinogenic polycholorinated biphenyls (PCBs) and dioxins. The fish oil makes salmon grow faster but also houses these fat-loving toxins.

One study* found that farmed salmon contains seven times more PCBs and dioxins than wild salmon. The highest levels were found in Scottish and Northern European farmed salmon, which account for only 7 percent of U.S. salmon. Chilean salmon is a better choice from the farmed salmon selections.

Salmon farmers are working to clean up their fish food, but in the meantime, it is good practice to follow these basic guidelines to avoid contaminants and maximize nutrients from your fish dish.

Try alternative varieties of farmed fish such as catfish and trout. These fish are less contaminated than farmed salmon and are also high in omega-3 oils. Look for wild salmon or salmon from organic

*Global Assessment of Organic Contaminants in Farmed Salmon. *Science*, v. 303, 9 January 2004.

farms. Organic fish encounter fewer pesticides, eat fish trimmings that are fit for humans, and live in less crowded pens. Cooking techniques to help minimize chemical exposure are to trim off fat (chemicals accumulate in fat) and to score, broil, or grill fish so that the juice drips off. You will still get plenty of the healthy omega-3 fish oil. Remove the skin before eating.

Ask at restaurants if the salmon is wild. All Alaskan salmon is wild, as is most canned salmon (a good calcium source, too). The best wild salmon varieties are coho, pink, and chum.

Don't be scared out of the water! Omega-3 oils in salmon and other fish offer us much greater cardiovascular and developmental benefits versus the relatively minimal risk of cancer.

Visit www.eatwellguide.org for organic food delivery or stores near you.

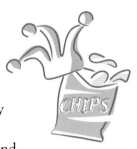

Foolish fats

Babies' developing bodies and brains are picky when it comes to the types of fats they need for healthy growth. Keep these pointers in mind when preparing your little one's menu.

Low-fat and fat-free products

No servings: birth to twenty-four months
Brains and nerves require fat to work properly. Babies need fat to build healthy nervous systems. Our brains are 60 percent fat!

Partially hydrogenated (trans) fats

Breast-feeding moms, all babies, and everyone else should completely avoid or at least minimize eating this type of fat. Trans-fats are commercially altered fats used to increase product shelf life. They interfere with fetal and post-birth natural fatty acid production essential to growth and nerve development. Trans-fat consumption also increases the risk of heart disease and diabetes.

Bistro basic

Be a "CLR" (Compulsive Label Reader)! These fats love to hang out in bakery foods, breads, snacks, and margarines. Labels may claim "zero trans-fats" if the serving size contains less than 0.5 grams, so double-check ingredients for "partially hydrogenated" oils.

Funky fruits

Not all fruits are created equally with regard to your baby's maturing digestive and immune systems. Certain fruits, though palate pleasing, may be a bit bothersome for your baby.

Citrus, berries, and tropical fruits

Allergies to berries, citrus, and certain tropical fruits such as kiwi, papaya, and mango are less common than the Big Eight food allergens, but they may be problematic for a small percentage of infants. Exercise caution when introducing these fruits, offering one at a time every few days. Start your baby with other healthy, less allergenic fruits such as bananas, apples, pears, peaches, cantaloupe, and apricots. Although there are no specific guidelines for when to introduce berries, citrus, and tropical fruit, it may be prudent to play it safe and wait until your baby is one year old.

Allergy alert!

If there is a strong family history of allergy or your baby has already displayed allergic sensitivities, avoid or be watchful for allergic symptoms for the first twenty-four months when you include these fruits on the menu!

Hold the honey . . . and the corn syrup

No servings: birth to twelve months
Honey and corn syrup may contain botulism spores, which release toxins that can overpower your baby's immature digestive system and may result in death.

Meat monsters

Meat is an excellent source of protein and iron. However, some meats also host certain chemical preservatives, bacteria, or risk for some types of cancer. If you like an occasional plate of meat and potatoes, take note of the following omnivore tips before you purée a little side dish for your baby.

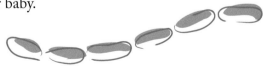

Hot dogs and ready-to-eat packaged luncheon or deli meats

No servings: birth to twenty-four months
Besides being not very nutritious, these meats may contain *listeria* bacteria that can attack babies' vulnerable immune systems. Meats freshly sliced at the deli are OK, such as fresh cuts of turkey or chicken.

Cured meats

No servings: birth to twenty-four months
Many of the cured meats, such as bacon, sausages, hot dogs, and some pre-packaged deli and lunch meats, contain preservatives called sodium nitrites or nitrates. High cooking temperatures can convert nitrites into cancer-causing substances. Look for healthier options in poultry or soy-based sausages and freshly roasted, packaged deli slices.

Be a CLR for nitrites or nitrates on labels. Certified organic meat products do not contain nitrites. However, even naturally cured meats are high in sodium, which is another reason to ration these foods. (See Appendix 2, Shopping for six to eight months, p. 126.)

Red meat

Servings: not more than twice a week when introducing meats, usually around seven months
Red meat may increase risk for future colon or pancreatic cancers. Limit this dish on your menu! If you plan to serve a beef recipe, try to select whole, boneless cuts of organic, grass-fed brands or beef from trusted cattle farms for a better quality meat.

Nut notes

A bite of peanut butter and jelly may seem to you the perfect first food, but the news on nuts is to take baby steps when introducing them to your newborn.

Tree nuts and peanuts

No servings: birth to twenty-four months

Nuts are a good source of protein, minerals, and healthy fats. However, tree nuts, peanuts, and nut butters and seeds, including tahini, are common food allergens. If your baby is not at risk for allergies, you may try offering small tastes of nuts such as peanuts or almond butter. Watch carefully to see if your baby shows any symptoms of allergy. Check your condiments closely; nuts may be hiding in foods like pesto and hummus.

Allergy alert!

If your family has a strong history of allergies, or your baby has already shown allergic sensitivities, avoid or use extreme caution when offering nuts and nut butters for the first three years. When dining out, always ask if the meal contains nuts! Beware of serving utensils that are shared with dishes that contain nuts. Even 1/10,000 of a teaspoon of nuts can trigger an allergic reaction in allergy-prone infants. For a listing of foods recalled due to possible nut contamination, check www.foodallergy.org/alerts.

Opt for organic

Many parents wonder if organic foods are really the best choice for feeding babies. Eating organically is healthy for all ages but is especially important for developing newborns.

100 percent certified organic foods

Start serving: at introduction of solid foods!
Pesticides keep the pesky bugs away but also may interfere with your baby's ability to absorb nutrients from foods, which puts normal growth and development at risk. In addition, some conventional fruits and vegetables have been shown to contain fewer vitamins and minerals than their organic counterparts. According to the National Academy of Sciences, 50 percent of lifetime pesticide exposure occurs during the first five years of life.

Babies may be more vulnerable to pesticides than adults for several reasons:

- **Babies eat more and drink more in proportion to their body weight compared to adults.**
- **Babies eat a more limited diet.**
- **Babies may distribute and filter toxins differently than adults, which could put normal hormonal, brain, and growth development at risk.**

Organic food may be a better choice, but truly ANY fruit and veggie is better than none! Follow these Bistro Basics to minimize pesticide or contaminant exposure:

Wash and scrub all fruits and veggies using warm water and a little liquid dish soap or store-brand fruit and vegetable washes.
Wash produce with rinds like cantaloupes to prevent your cutting knife from transferring pesticides and bacteria into the fruit.
Remove outer leaves and break apart broccoli or cauliflower before washing.

Serve a wide variety of produce.
Buy seasonally or locally grown foods (less spraying and wax
 coating).
Trim fats from meat, poultry, and fish (fatty tissue attracts
 chemicals).
Wash can lids before opening the cans.

If organic edibles are emptying your wallet, spend selectively on the
items below and look for less costly frozen organic brands.

Save some grocery money by buying conventional brands from the
 Conventional Keepers foods and spend a little extra on organic
 brands from the foods in the Dirty Dozen.

The Dirty Dozen	Conventional Keepers
(highest pesticide residues)	(lowest pesticide residues)
Apples	Asparagus
Bell peppers	Avocados
Cherries	Bananas
Celery	Broccoli
Imported grapes	Cauliflower
Peaches	Kiwi
Pears	Mangos
Potatoes	Onions
Nectarines	Papaya
Red raspberries	Pineapple
Spinach	Sweet corn
Strawberries	Sweet peas

The more we demand organic foods, the more affordable they become! Look for the USDA "100% Certified Organic" seal on foods. Check www.consumersunion.org for updates. For organic food delivery or stores near you, check www.eatwellguide.org/search.cfm.

Plastic priorities

Plastics have their place in our world but not in the world of your newborn. Synthetic chemical compounds such as bisphenol A and dioxins in some plastics provide benefits for product structure and durability. However, health problems arise when those materials are used in food and beverage containers or wraps and the chemicals migrate from plastic to food to people!

Scientists are concerned about animal studies that show these types of chemicals interfering with normal hormone and nervous system function as well as increasing the risk for certain cancers. During fetal, infant, and child stages of rapid growth, these effects could alter the course of normal brain and behavioral development.

How do you protect your baby from potentially harmful plasticizers? Follow these Bistro Basics:

If you bottle-feed your baby, choose glass bottles or plastic bottles that are BPA-free.

Make sure that your baby food storage containers and canned foods are BPA-free. Foods packaged in cardboard cartons, glass, or pouches are safer alternatives. If you use infant formula, powdered rather than canned liquid formulas reduce exposure to BPA.

When you store leftovers, leave an inch or more space between the food and the plastic wrap. Use glass containers or food storage baggies, repackage plastic-wrapped grocery foods or takeout, and throw away old plastic containers.

Microwave foods in microwave-safe glass, Corning ware, or ceramic, and cover containers with paper towels, parchment paper, or wax paper. Never microwave in takeout containers, plastic food tubs, plastic storage bags, grocery bags, or used microwave dinner containers. Put frozen meals in microwave-safe dishes to defrost.

Check www.niehs.nih.gov/health for more information and www. ewg.org for a guide to baby-safe bottles.

Skip the salt, sugar, and spices

No servings: birth to twenty-four months
Adding salt causes babies' developing kidneys to work overtime and can promote future salt cravings. The estimated minimum amount of salt that a six- to eleven-month-old infant needs is 200 milligrams per day.

One teaspoon of salt = 2,300 milligrams!

Adding sugar and offering sugary foods increase chances for diarrhea and dental decay. Think of sugar as "empty calories" that take space away from more nutrient-dense foods.

Babies have more taste buds than adults, which increases their sensitivity to flavors. Pouring on the spices may promote allergies and cause a dependency on

certain tastes. Depending
on family customs and what
you eat during pregnancy and
while breast-feeding, babies'
preferences for spices vary.
Try mild spices such as cinnamon, ginger,
vanilla, or mint rather than jalapeño!

Bistro basic

Let babies get used to life
before adding the spice to it!

Vexing veggies

Yes, vegetables are an excellent source of nutrition and are wonderful
first foods for babies. However, a few foods from the plant kingdom
should be postponed until later stages.

Home-prepared or canned spinach, beets, turnips, carrots, or collard greens

No servings: birth to six months
Home-prepared baby foods from fresh, frozen, or canned brands
of spinach, beets, turnips, carrots, or collard greens may pose a
health risk for newborns less than six months of
age. These types of veggies contain nitrates—
chemicals that can cause a blood condition
called methemoglobinemia, where not enough
oxygen can reach body tissues. Nitrate content
in veggies relates to sun exposure, crop location,
groundwater, and fertilizers. Organic brands may
also contain nitrates.

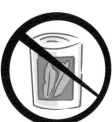

Serving baby food brands of these vegetables is fine.

Canned vegetables of any variety

No servings: birth to twenty-four months
Watch the salt (sodium)! Canned vegetables as well as other canned foods are typically very high in sodium, which acts as a preservative to prolong the shelf life of food. Labels on cans indicating "no salt added" or frozen vegetables are better alternatives.

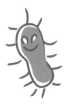

Raw sprouts

No servings
Raw sprouts may contain *Salmonella*, *E. coli*, and the canavanine toxin.

Watch the wheat

The protein in wheat, called "gluten," is an allergen. If your baby is genetically prone to allergy or has already shown allergic sensitivities, hold off or use caution in serving whole-wheat bakery foods, pastas, and cereals during the first year. If your baby has no family history of allergy, you may try offering small tastes of wheat breads, cereals, and pastas, but watch carefully for any allergic reaction.

Allergy alert!
Oats, barley, kamut, spelt, kasha, rye, bulgur, bran, wheat germ, einkorn, emmer, durum flour, graham, malt, matzo meal, seitan, and semolina also contain gluten. Discuss excluding these foods from your baby's diet with your pediatrician if your baby has a family history of celiac disease. Wheat may be in white breads and pastas as well as in the brown varieties.

Check www.celiac.org for gluten-free products.

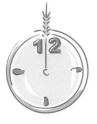

Celiac sprue is an autoimmune gastrointestinal disorder also triggered by gluten and interferes with nutrient absorption. Babies with a genetic predisposition may be more at risk of developing celiac disease if they are exposed to wheat too soon.

Shopping smarts

Grocery shopping can be quite overwhelming, especially with a baby on board. I realize that I may be alone in my love of spending hours in the store staring at hundreds of food labels and that you would probably prefer to enter and exit as quickly as possible. I have asked parents whether they want general guidelines of what to look for at the market or if they simply want to be told which are the best brands to buy. The majority answered, "Just tell us what to buy!"

So, I decided to do both. Thousands of brands are out there and are constantly evolving. Some companies offer wonderful products but are only distributed regionally. It is nearly impossible to list all of the good brands, so here's some help for narrowing your food search. The following tips offer general guidelines on how to navigate the grocery maze and choose healthy foods. For some specific brand suggestions, visit Baby Bistro Appendix 2, p. 125.

Shopping trip tips

For easy shopping, make your list according to the aisles in your favorite market. Keep your list in an accessible spot like on the refrigerator so that you can add to it as the thought pops into your head. You'll forget two seconds later!

Baby food brands usually have "primary" or #1 on the label to indicate first baby foods, "secondary" or #2 on second-stage foods, and #3 for third-stage foods. Most labels also list the appropriate age range for that particular food item.

Opt for organic! Check the frozen section for organic fruits and veggies. They are less expensive and will not spoil, so they can be used as needed.

Add meats, fish, and frozen foods to your cart last to maximize freshness.

Buy whole-fat dairy items for your baby through two years of age.

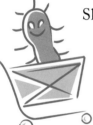

Shop for extra frozen favorites to store with grandparents or anywhere you visit frequently.

Keep a small, antiseptic spray handy for dirty grocery carts that your baby may want to taste!

Practice your "CLR" (Compulsive Label Reader) skills and do your best to avoid the following ingredients:

- **Trans-fats (partially hydrogenated fats)**
- **Hydrogenated oils, lard, palm kernel oil, coconut oils, shortening, and beef tallow (in the top three ingredients)**
- **Saturated fat (more than three grams per serving)**
- **Sodium (more than 140 milligrams per serving)**

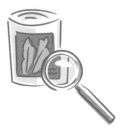

- Sugar, high-fructose corn syrup (HFCS), fructose, honey, glucose, and sucrose (in the top three ingredients)
- Food additives: nitrates, nitrites, sulfites, and artificial flavoring or coloring

If your baby has food allergies, check labels to see if the food contains any allergy-related ingredient. Albumin (egg), casein (milk), and gluten (wheat) are allergenic proteins from foods. The Food Allergen Consumer Protection Act instructs companies to clearly list on food labels whether the product is made with milk, eggs, peanuts, tree nuts, wheat, soy, shellfish, or fish.

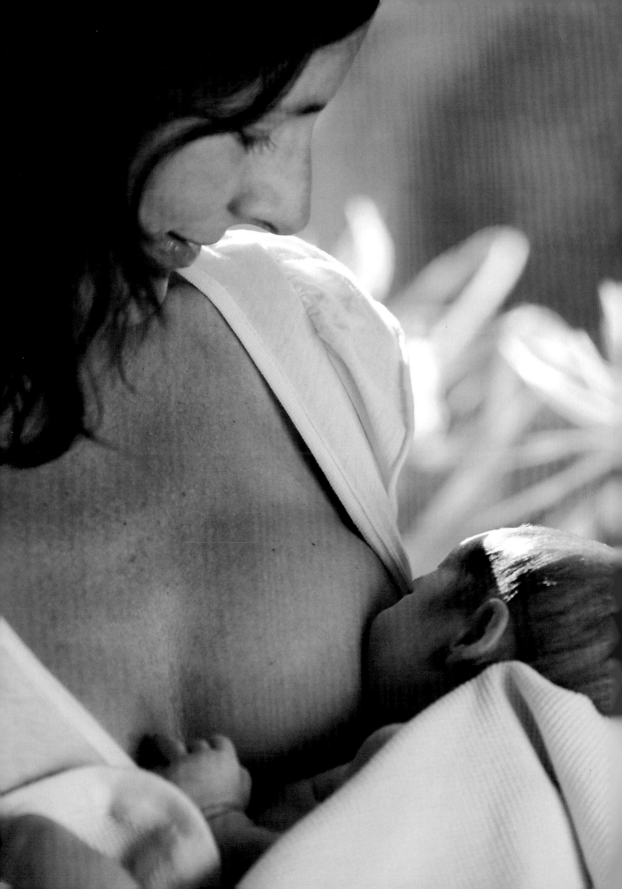

Entrées

Birth to four months

You may be thinking, what in the world is she talking about with "entrées" during the birth to four-month stage? Newborn babies can't eat solid foods! You are absolutely right, but your baby is certainly going to be demanding very frequent meals from your "open twenty-four hours" baby bistro!

The menu is simple during this stage of infancy. Your repeat daily special is breast milk or an iron-fortified formula, which offers all of the nutrition that healthy babies require. This chapter will help you progress from beginner to master chef in feeding your baby during the first months of life.

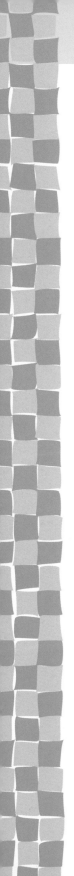

Nutrient needs

This chart is just an FYI (For Your Information), not an FYO (Freak You Out)!

If your baby is feeding normally, your breast milk or a quality formula will do the trick!

Recommended calorie, protein, and fat intake for birth to four months			
Pounds	Calories/Day	Protein(g)/Day	Fat(g)/Day
5	275	3	11
7	350	5	16
9	430	6	21
11	510	8	25
13	590	10	30
15	670	12	34
17	750	14	39
20	870	17	46

Your baby should gain one to two pounds per month and reach twice its birth weight by four to six months. Premature babies or babies with some type of metabolic disorder may have special needs. Check with your health care provider!

Breast milk

The American Academy of Pediatrics (AAP) recommends breast-feeding exclusively from birth to six months. Research shows that breast-feeding for a longer duration boosts immunity and decreases your baby's risk for ear infections, allergies, asthma, diabetes, and obesity. Breast-feeding may also protect moms from future risk of certain cancers and osteoporosis.

Preparation and serving suggestions for the "Milkmom"

Drink six to eight glasses of fluid every day. Practice drinking a glass each time you breast-feed.

Eat about 200 calories per day more than you did during pregnancy. Try to make healthy, nutrient-dense snacks your habit. These extra calories are not an excuse to give in to every French fry or candy craving!

Make sure that you get enough protein, calcium, and B vitamins, and continue your prenatal supplement and DHA.

Chef's suggestions

Do not supplement breast milk or formula by mixing cereals and other solids into the bottle. Until about six months, your baby's digestive system is not ready for much more than milk. You may think of them as little side dishes, but extra solids add too many calories; may cause allergies, constipation, or dislike of certain tastes; and may increase the risk for diabetes and obesity. Slipping in solids will not necessarily help babies with acid reflux, sleeping longer, or spitting up either!

If your baby keeps ordering seconds, step up the feedings and get out the next size of clothing! Growth spurts occur around two weeks, six to eight weeks, three months, and six months.

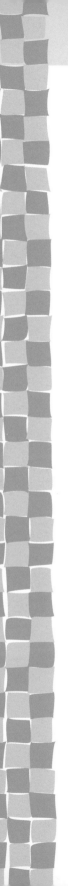

Nurse on demand, usually every two to three hours (20 to 27 ounces or 600 to 800 milliliters per day). Your body will keep up with extra orders from your baby during growth spurts.

Breathe and relax during feeding times. This is a special bonding time for you and your baby.

Taste test

Spicy foods can change the taste of your breast milk in a way that your baby may or may not appreciate. If you eat spicy foods regularly, your baby will probably be fine with the flavor of your breast milk after a tears-in-your-eyes, tongue-fanning Thai takeout meal. If your milk special of the day gets sent back to the kitchen, however, try a more bland meal before breast-feeding.

Lactic acid buildup from exercise may also change the taste of breast milk. Waiting one hour after exercise to breast-feed allows lactic acid to normalize.

Quality checks

Limit alcoholic drinks and avoid smoking. If you choose to have a drink, do so after breast-feeding, not before. Alcohol clears from breast milk as it is cleared from the bloodstream (one ounce per hour). "Pumping and dumping" will not rid your breast milk of alcohol if you do not wait the appropriate time to breast-feed after a drink (three hours for five ounces of wine or twelve ounces of beer). Research indicates that small amounts of alcohol interfere with infant sleep patterns. Excessive drinking by nursing moms may cause developmental disabilities.

If you have a family history of food allergies, be aware of your baby's reaction after you eat those types of foods. If your baby shows discomfort after you eat certain foods, you may need to exclude them from your diet. Common foods that trigger a reaction in some babies are eggs, wheat, dairy, tree nuts, peanuts, shellfish, and soy. Other foods that occasionally may pose a problem are cruciferous veggies like broccoli and cauliflower, onions, bell peppers, or garlic. Cooking your vegetables rather than eating them raw may be less irritating. Take note of the food(s) you think bother your baby and discuss your options with your health care provider.

Keep your carton-brand milk consumption to about two cups per day. Overconsumption may overload your breast milk with protein and salt.

Sleep-deprived moms may welcome back their beloved coffee, but that does not equate to hourly triple espresso shots! Caffeine transfers into breast milk in very small amounts. Keep your caffeine consumption at 100 to 200 milligrams per day (one regular cup of coffee equals 100 milligrams). Studies have shown interrupted sleep patterns, nervousness, poor feeding, and irritability in infants whose mothers drink more than 300 milligrams of caffeinated beverages per day.

Low levels of nutrients in your diet affect the quantity, not the quality, of breast milk. Your body sacrifices its own nutrient stores to deliver nutritious milk to your baby.

Nutrients in breast milk that are most sensitive to your diet are vitamins A, B12, E, D, and selenium. Even though you are operating on three hours of sleep and have lost all memory-recall skills, make the effort to eat, and make it nutritious! Continue taking your prenatal multivitamin to help cover any dietary nutrition gaps.

Antioxidant levels in breast milk drop with refrigeration, freezing, and heating. You may freeze breast milk at 0°F (-19°C) for up to six months or refrigerate it at 32°F to 40°F (0°C to 5°C) for up to eight days. Freeze it in glass or hard-sided plastic containers and defrost it in warm water.

Delete artificial trans fats from your diet! These fats are unhealthy and pass into breast milk.

Speaking of diet, do not start one while breast-feeding. Here is your best excuse ever to procrastinate a little longer. You will risk your baby's health as well as your own if you diet. You should naturally drop pregnancy pounds with breast-feeding.

Don't got milk? Try . . . a galactagogue!

This a fancy word for something that promotes the flow of milk, and no, beer is not an effective method! Although none are FDA approved or scientifically proven, they have been used safely and with some success. Check with your health care provider if you decide to try a galactagogue, and report any reaction. The strongest promoters of milk are rest, good diet, plenty of fluids, and your own baby sucking!

Some common galactagogues are:

- Anise
- Borage
- Cumin
- Dill
- Fennel
- Fenugreek
- Oatmeal
- Nettle

You may notice a maple syrup odor in your sweat and urine with fenugreek.

You can find these in health food or specialty markets in the form of supplements, tea, or seeds. Borage may also be purchased as oil.

Medications and breast-feeding

The American Academy of Pediatrics (AAP) has classified drugs relating to breast-feeding into seven categories, from highly dangerous to those that are safe and compatible. If you have any questions regarding medications, ask your health care provider.

1. Cytotoxic (cell killer) drugs, such as chemotherapy drugs

2. Drugs of abuse, like cocaine or heroin, which can harm and be addictive to babies

3. Radioactive drugs from radiation treatment, which require a temporary stop in breast-feeding

4. Drugs that may be of concern, but the effects on nursing infants are unknown, including anti-anxiety drugs and anti-depressants

5. Drugs to use with caution, such as lithium, aspirin, or primidone, where significant effects have been associated with some nursing infants

6. Drugs that are usually compatible with nursing, such as acetaminophen, many antibiotics, anti-epileptics, most antihistamines, most antihypertensives, codeine, decongestants, ibuprofen, insulin, quinine, warfarin, thyroid medications, moderate alcohol, and moderate caffeine

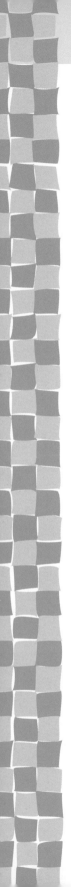

7. Food and environmental agents such as aspartame, chocolate, lead, mercury, monosodium glutamate, or vegetarian diets

Breast implants, herbals, and smoking

Silicon and saline breast implants are not considered a risk to breast-fed infants. Most women with breast implants are able to breast-feed normally.

Herbal supplements and nicotine are not listed within the seven drug categories. Smoking is discouraged but not prohibited. Breast-feeding is still considered best for your baby's health. Remember that smoking will put your baby at risk for delayed weight gain, infections (i.e. ear), SIDS, asthma, and lung damage.

Useful resources

www.fda.gov/medwatch
To learn about new drug safety research and adverse reactions.

http://pediatrics.aappublications.org
The transfer of drugs and other chemicals into human milk. *Pediatrics*, Vol. 108, No. 3, September 2001, pp. 776-789.

Lactation Study Center at the University of Rochester
(585) 275-0088. The Lactation Study Center is a resource for medical professionals. Your health care provider can call for you to access more information on your medication.

Formula fundamentals . . . Menu choices

There are many reasons why you may choose to feed your baby formula. Some women are physically unable to breast-feed, their baby may be premature and may need extra nutrition, or they adopted their precious little one. Whatever the reason, rest assured that excellent infant formulas are available on the market, and they continue to improve. Here are the general categories of baby formulas from which you may choose with the help of your pediatrician.

Standard cow's milk–based formula

This type of formula is the most common. It contains lactose (the sugar in milk) and intact or partially hydrolyzed (predigested) milk protein (casein). Choose a formula containing iron, DHA and ARA. DHA and ARA are two fatty acids found in breast milk that are vital to infant cognitive and visual development. Formulas that also include "friendly bacteria" cultures known as probiotics offer additional health benefits and more closely resemble breast milk.

Bistro Bests These are my favorite formulas for normal, healthy infants. They are widely available and are the most similar to natural breast milk. Because formulas continue to evolve and some infants have special needs, discuss your formula options with your health care provider.

Bright Beginnings Organic with Lipids
Enfamil Lipil with Iron
Nestle Good Start Natural Cultures
Similac Organic DHA and ARA

Soy-based formula

Soy formulas are alternatives for vegan infants and for infants diagnosed with galactosemia or lactose intolerance (extremely rare) whose moms cannot breast-feed. Forty-three percent of infants with a cow's milk allergy develop allergies to soy formulas as well; therefore, a hypoallergenic formula is a better choice for those babies who have dairy allergies. Soy formulas do support normal growth and development, and in nearly a century of use, no adverse effects on infant hormonal status have been observed from the phytoestrogens (plant hormones) in soy.

Hypoallergenic formula

This type of formula is the best choice for non-vegan babies who have a milk allergy. You will see two kinds on the labels:

1. Extensively hydrolyzed protein or "protein hydrosylate." This is cow's milk protein that is partially broken down, such as in Alimentum or Nutramigen.
2. Free amino acid-based. These contain no whole proteins, such as in Neocate.

Lactose-free formula

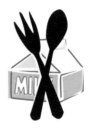

This formula does not contain the milk sugar, lactose. Lactose-intolerant babies are extremely rare!

Specialized formula

These formulas are for premies or for infants who have specific metabolic disorders.

For families serving formula, The American Academy of Pediatrics (AAP) recommends iron-fortified formulas (4 to 12 milligrams per liter) for all infants from birth to twelve months. There is no evidence that the amount of iron in baby formula causes constipation.

Formula serving suggestions

Whether you and your baby are just beginners or you just need a brush up, the following formula preparation and feeding tips should help you reach expert status in no time.

- Feed on demand.
- Expect to serve between 20 to 27 ounces (600 to 800 milliliters) per day.
- Boil unfiltered water for powder formulas for a full five minutes to sterilize.
- Avoid propping up the bottle during feeding.
- Throw out leftovers! The bacteria from your baby's mouth love to feast on the nutrients in leftover formula and will cause contamination.
- Do not water down formulas.
- Do not use low-iron formulas. Babies need iron for red blood cell formation and to prevent iron deficiency anemia.
- Notify your health care provider if you notice any of the following allergic reactions: diarrhea, rash, dry skin, wheezing, asthma, facial swelling, vomiting, or blood or mucus in the stool (generally indicates a cow milk allergy). You may need to switch formulas.
- Relax and enjoy feeding times. This is your time for you and your baby to bond.

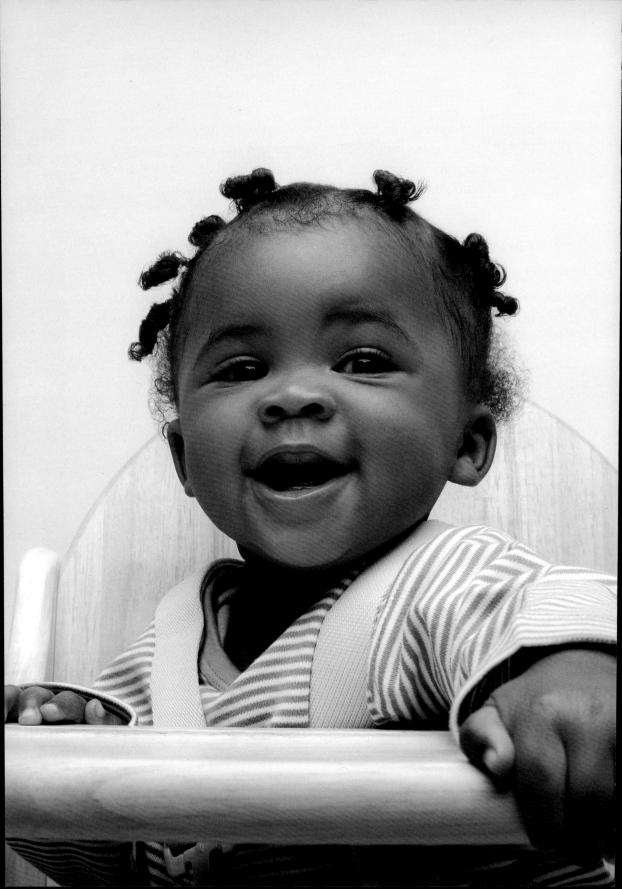

Entrées

Four to six months

This age stage is so much fun. You will see your baby begin to notice more the surrounding environment, flash you some smiles, unveil charm and personality, and start to show signs of readiness for trying some solid foods! Let's get you ready too, so that you know what to look for and how to approach this new, exciting stage of your baby's development.

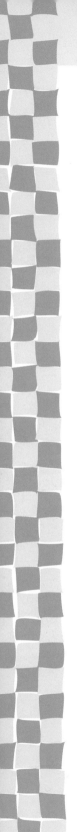

Nutrient needs

This chart is the same as the birth to four months nutrient needs chart. The difference is that now you may be supplying some of the nutrients from solid foods in addition to breast milk or formula.

Recommended calorie, protein, and fat intake for four to six months			
Pounds	Calories/Day	Protein(g)/Day	Fat(g)/Day
5	155	3	11
7	235	5	16
9	315	6	21
11	395	8	25
13	475	10	30
15	555	12	34
17	635	14	39
20	755	17	46

Check out the fat!

Fat equals almost half a day's calories! One gram of fat equals nine calories. Babies naturally require more fat for developing brains and growing bodies.

Your baby should gain one to two pounds per month and reach twice its birth weight by four to six months. Premature or other special-needs babies may have supplemental requirements such as for extra iron or calories. Check with your health care provider.

Signals for solids

Don't you just wish they could speak up and say, "Hello, I'm developmentally and physically ready to eat some solid food now?" Unfortunately, babies are 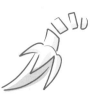 not that direct, but if you add up all the signs, it can be fairly obvious they are ready to try the next item on the menu.

Do you nurse about eight times per day or provide 900 milliliters or more of formula per day? Has your baby reached approximately twice its birth weight?

Is your baby . . .

teething?

sitting up?

controlling head movements?

making chewing motions?

watching what you are eating with increased interest?

moving its tongue from side to side and back and forth when food is in its mouth?

Check with your health care provider and don't stress about being on the same schedule as the books suggest. And don't pay attention to the schedule that your friends' babies are on. Watch your one-of-a-kind baby for signs of when the time is right for the solid stuff!

It is best to hold the solids until your baby is nearing six months of age. The AAP supports exclusive breast-feeding until babies are approximately six months old.

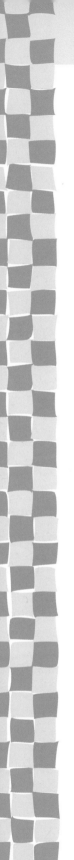

Serving suggestions for solids

Be slow to introduce new solids. You may be excited about your baby starting to eat real food, but you need to watch out for allergies. Add one new food every four to six days, watching for any reaction. Typical allergic reactions are rash, vomiting, diarrhea, facial swelling, wheezing, asthma, or blood or mucus in the stool. Blood in the stool usually indicates a cow milk allergy.

Which food first? Scientifically speaking, there is no rule for which food is best to start feeding your baby. Begin with foods that are easy to digest such as yellow or orange veggies, fruits, or gluten-free cereals. Sweet potatoes, bananas, or iron-fortified rice cereals are all safe and healthy options. Serve veggies before fruit to help avoid a sweet tooth! Iron-fortified rice cereal is a good starter food to protect against iron-deficiency anemia.

Begin by offering a little breast milk or formula to calm your hungry baby. If your baby wants to skip straight to solids, that is fine!

Using a baby spoon, place about one-fourth teaspoon of your purée of choice on your baby's tongue. Try to establish a routine of offering about one tablespoon of solids once or twice a day with breakfast or lunch, building to three times a day.

Think simple, keeping servings to single ingredients. Complicated food combinations make it difficult to determine which food is the culprit if your baby has an allergic reaction. Combining a variety of puréed foods is fine once you know your baby is not allergic to them.

Force-feeding is not a helpful practice. You may, however, need to be a little pushy with that first bite!

Try to keep distractions to a low volume.

Reserve the same dining location to establish a routine.

Make sure that your baby is snug and secure in a high chair during feeding times.

Feeding on demand is fine. Focus on nutrition; don't worry about when and how much.

Bistro basic

Sweeter later!
If both vegetables and fruit are on the menu, offer those appetizing veggie purées first, in case your baby decides to only eat the sweet stuff.

Avoid feeding your baby out of the baby food jar if you only use part of its contents. The bacteria from saliva grow in the leftovers and cause spoilage and germ overgrowth.

Leftovers can be saved in the fridge for up to two days.

Spitting out food is a normal reflex. It takes practice to eat, just like learning to ride a bike!

Foods that trouble you may also trouble your baby.

Offer some water in addition to breast milk or formula to avoid dehydration, especially if your baby has diarrhea.

Worry less!

Solids du Jour

Here are some possible menu additions for when your baby nears six months of age. All meals should be served with breast milk, iron-fortified formula, or soy formula for vegan clientele.

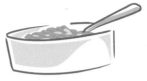

Iron-fortified rice cereal

This cereal is easiest to digest and is least likely to cause allergies for your young patrons. Rice cereal is also a daily essential (four or more dry tablespoons per day) to help prevent iron deficiency anemia. The consistency should be thin and creamy.

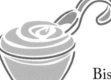

Plain, puréed vegetables

Bistro bests are sweet potatoes, pumpkins, squash varieties, carrots, asparagus, broccoli, spinach, green beans, split peas, green peas, and parsnips. Yellow veggies are easiest to digest except for corn. Wait until your baby has at least advanced to green veggies before serving a corn dish.

Plain, unsweetened, puréed fruits

The Bistro bests are cantaloupes, nectarines, peaches, apricots, avocadoes, bananas, pears, apples, plums, and watermelons.

Chef's secret

Bananas, nectarines, and peaches stain!

Solids from scratch . . . Try your hand at homemade

Skip adding extra sugar, salt, or strong spices. Plain food is plenty for babies!

Remove all strings, seeds, and skins from fruits and vegetables to prevent choking. To remove skins and seeds press the food through a sieve or use a baby-food grinder or food mill.

Meaty meals begin around seven to eight months. Slice and chop meats against the grain to avoid stringiness.

Wash and cook food thoroughly.

Make extra food and save it for later dishes!

Chef's secret

Root veggies such as sweet potatoes are easy to cook in the microwave on root setting; you can then purée or mash them. Don't forget to poke holes in the skin to avoid having your mash all over the inside of the microwave!

Safe storage

Refrigerate baby food for up to two days only.

Freeze purées and blends in ice cube trays enclosed in a freezer bag. Empty frozen cubes into another freezer bag and store fruits or veggies up to six months and meats up to two months. Don't forget to write the date on the bag! Now you'll have home-cooked, easy, meal-size servings just a freezer away. Thaw frozen purées in the fridge or saucepan. Allow reheated food to cool, then stir and finger test it to make sure that the temperature is even and lukewarm.

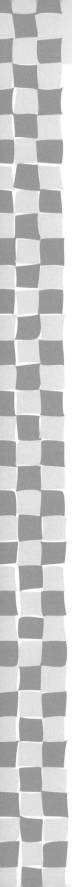

When you are defrosting your carefully prepared cubes of purée, it is helpful to know how much to defrost for a typical serving size for babies:

one ice cube equals one ounce

one jar of baby food equals three to four ounces

Purées

Food processors, blenders, and baby-food grinders or food mills can be used to make purées. Food processors are handy to purée large batches and freeze for later. Baby-food grinders or small food processors are fabulous for preparing smaller portions of whatever baby-edible specials you have made for dinner or have left over in the fridge.

To prepare a purée, first lightly steam or microwave the veggies to retain most of their nutrients. Blend them to a thin, smooth, creamy consistency. Defrosted fibrous veggies such as broccoli or carrots do not grind or purée as well as when they are freshly cooked. Starchier defrosted veggies like peas prove to be a better purée!

To save time, purée the baby-edible foods you prepared for your meal.

You can thin purées with any broth, breast milk, or formula, or you can use the left-over water from cooking the veggies.

Bistro recipes . . . Purées

Smashing winter squash
MAKES 3–4 OUNCES

- ½ winter squash (acorn, butternut)

Remove seeds from squash and bake, microwave, or steam until tender. Scoop out flesh and pass through food mill or blend in food processor.

Peas please!
MAKES 3–4 OUNCES

- 1 cup frozen organic peas

Steam peas on stove or in microwave. Purée with food mill or food processor.

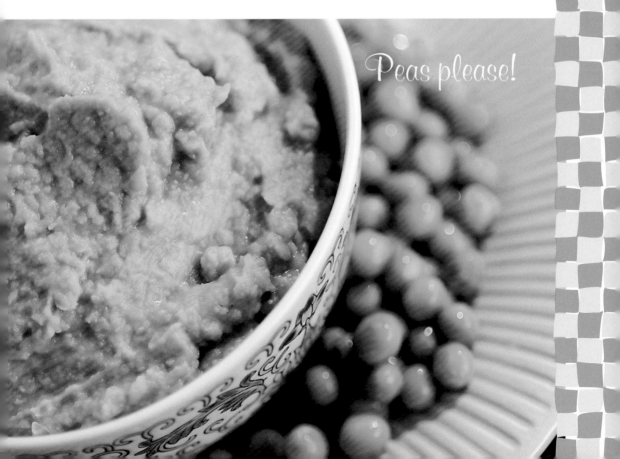

Peas please!

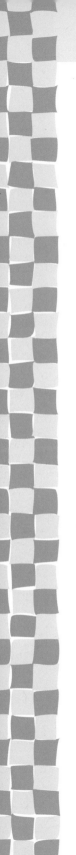

Cantaloupe soup

MAKES 8–12 OUNCES

- 1 ripe organic cantaloupe

Peel and remove seeds from cantaloupe. Cut into chunks and blend in food processor. *(See photo on opposite page.)*

Freeze extras in ice cube tray.

Purely pears

MAKES 3–4 OUNCES

- 1 ripe organic pear

Cut and core the pear. If you're using a food processor, remove the skin. Food mills or baby-food grinders will separate the skin from the purée.

Purée! Three to four pears will fill your ice cube tray.

Quick peach purée

MAKES 4–6 OUNCES

- 1 can unsweetened, plain organic peaches or 1½ cups frozen organic peach slices, thawed

Purée and serve!

All about applesauce

MAKES 12 OUNCES

- 4 medium-size apples of any variety, peeled and chopped

Cover and simmer gently, stirring occasionally for about 20 minutes until tender.

Purée in food mill or food processor.

Cantaloupe soup

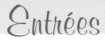

Simply sweet potatoes

MAKES 8 OUNCES

- 1 sweet potato
- 6 tablespoons veggie broth
- 1 teaspoon olive oil

Poke holes in the sweet potato and microwave to cook until soft.
Peel off skin and purée with the rest of the ingredients. *(See photo on opposite page.)*

Add ½ cup plain, organic, whole fat yogurt as a delicious twist for babies more than seven moths old.

Baby carrot purée*

MAKES 3-4 OUNCES

- 1 cup fresh organic baby carrots

Steam over stove or in microwave. Purée in food processor or food mill.

*Not for babies less than six months old

Simply sweet potatoes

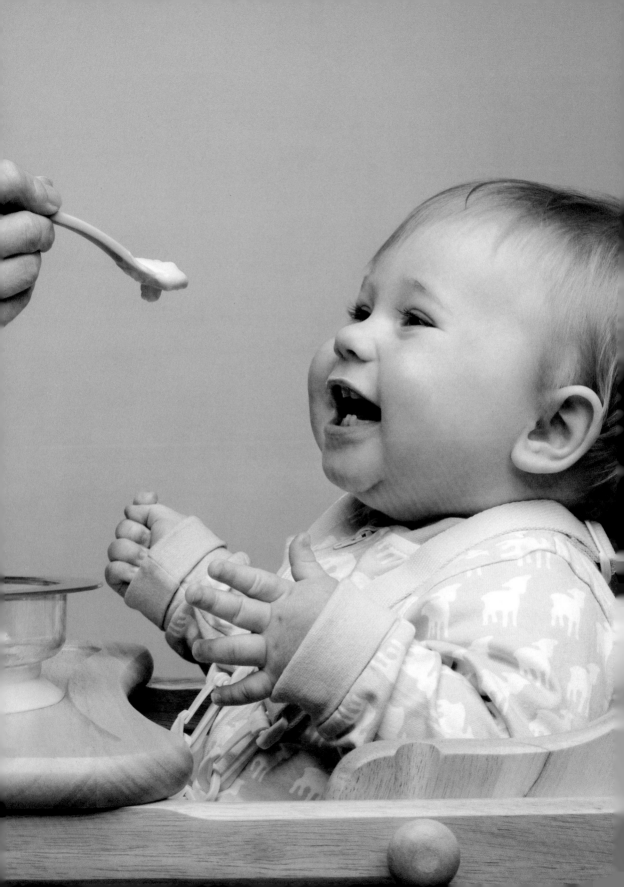

Entrées

Six to eight months

How did six months fly by so quickly? As you and your baby are rounding that half-year mark, the prospect of feeding solid food is no longer on the horizon. You have been coasting along with breast-feeding or formula-feeding when suddenly that old-shoe comfort changes into confusion as you ponder questions like which foods are nutritious and safe to feed my baby, when do I offer them, and how much?

If they haven't already tasted some first foods, most babies at this age make it quite obvious they want something new on the menu. Some cultures traditionally place their native foods on babies' tongues so that they will like the foods and will work hard to cultivate them when they grow up. Unless you farm for a living, your only concern is which foods will help your baby grow! This chapter covering six to eight months of age will help you feel confident in entering this new, exciting, and messy stage of feeding your little one.

Nutrient needs

This table is different from the first two nutrient needs tables that cover birth to six months. The calorie and protein needs are slightly less, fat is still 30 to 54 percent of calories, and weight gain is expected to drop to a half to one pound per month.

Calorie, protein, and fat intake for six to eight months			
Pounds	Calories/Day	Protein(g)/Day	Fat(g)/Day
15	520	8	22
17	600	9	25
19	680	10	28
21	760	11	31
23	840	12	34
25	920	14	37
27	1,000	15	40
30	1,120	16	45

Premature or other special-needs babies may have supplemental requirements. Check with your health care provider.

62

> **Check out the fat!**
> Fat equals almost half a day's calories! Babies need fat for brain and central nervous system development and for their growing bodies.
> **1 gram = 9 calories**

Serving suggestions

Iron is an absolute necessity. By six months of age, babies have tapped out their iron stores from birth and need extra iron in addition to breast milk or formula. Meats and beans offer the most, but babies need to wait until seven or eight months of age to choose those foods from the menu.

For now, select iron-rich fruits, veggies, and other iron-rich foods.

Fruits: cantaloupes, pears, watermelons, dried fruits (very sweet, use sparingly!), avocadoes

Veggies: butternut squash, pumpkins, broccoli, spinach, beets

Other iron-rich foods: iron-fortified rice cereals, millet, quinoa, amaranth, nutritional yeast, blackstrap molasses

Vary or combine the fruit and veggie entrées once you know your baby is not allergic to them.

Adjust textured foods according to dental maturity. Anything can be ground or puréed!

Try mixing one to two tablespoons of rice cereal into purées for extra nutrition and a creamier texture.

Remember the "Sweeter Later" rule! For seven- to eight-month-olds, cool hot cereals with a dollop of plain yogurt.

Introducing . . . the sippy cup! Try offering one with some water.

Encourage self-feeding with finger foods for a guaranteed mess, fun, and freedom for the chef! Dogs are great mobile mops!

Second servings for seven- to eight-month-old diners

First foods are like the first course of fine dining. They should be light and open the palate to other flavors. Once your baby is accustomed to your selection of appetizers from the cereal, fruit, and vegetable groups, you may begin to introduce some more complex protein sources at around seven to eight months of age.

Choose from these options:

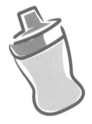

- Assorted meats
- Assorted meat alternatives
- Fish (see First Course, Fishy Fish, p. 17)
- Cheeses
- Cheese alternatives
- Whole-fat plain yogurts
- Nondairy yogurts
- Beans

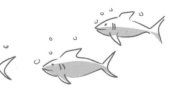

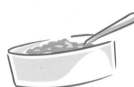

Chef's suggestions

Grind, purée, mash, or finely chop foods depending on your baby's ability to chew lumpier blends. Don't wait too long to introduce texture into smooth purées! You want to encourage your baby's chewing development. Watch for allergic reactions when introducing soy-based foods (see First Course, Allergy Advice, p. 10).

More on the menu

As executive chef, you are always looking for dishes that are appetizing yet developmentally appropriate for your V.I.B.P. (Very Important Baby Patron). This is a fun time when you can experiment with creamy cereals, combination purées, and mashes that even a grown-up would eat. Of course, you can't tell them it is "baby food." All meals may be served with breast milk, iron-fortified formula, or iron-fortified soy formula for vegan clientele.

Cereal symphony

Choose from some of these iron-rich cereals. Iron-fortified rice cereal is a great starter food for babies but is not the only option. If your baby rejects rice cereal or you simply want to try something different, whip up one of the following easy-to-digest, nutrient-packed porridges.

Cooking times:

Iron-fortified baby rice cereal	3 to 5 minutes
Rolled oats or barley flakes	3 to 5 minutes
Short-grain brown or white rice	15 minutes for instant 50 minutes for traditional
Quinoa	15 minutes (rinse first to remove bitter flavor)
Amaranth	25 to 30 minutes
Millet	30 to 35 minutes

Chef's secret

If you are feeling adventurous, try amaranth, quinoa, or millet. These "ancient grains" are great sources of iron and protein and are free of gluten (the protein allergen in wheat). Some African cultures commonly serve millet gruels mixed with mashed bananas as a first food to complement breast-feeding. You can find these grains in the hot cereal section of most large markets or health food stores.

Try flavoring cereals by cooking with one or two of the following: chopped dried or fresh fruit, or one teaspoon of vanilla, maple syrup, molasses, or cinnamon. Dried fruit and molasses add an extra boost of iron. Cool cereals by stirring in a little applesauce or plain yogurt.

Chef's tip

Simmering cereal grains on the old-fashioned stove is actually easier to monitor than the microwave. Prepare a big batch for the week to have ready for hungry babies!

Easy creamy rice porridge   MAKES EIGHT 2 OUNCE SERVINGS

- 1 cup cooked brown or white short-grain rice
- 2 tablespoons unsweetened applesauce
- 1½ cups water

Combine rice and water in small saucepan and bring to boil. Simmer 10 to 15 minutes until thick with a creamy consistency, stirring occasionally. Stir in applesauce.

Apple cinnamon amaranth   MAKES 2–3 SERVINGS

- ¼ cup cooked amaranth
- 1 tablespoon chopped raisins
- 2 tablespoons water
- sprinkle of cinnamon
- ¼ teaspoon vanilla
- 1 tablespoon unsweetened applesauce

Mix first five ingredients in small glass bowl. Microwave on high for 2 minutes. Remove and stir in applesauce to cool. You may substitute cooked rice, quinoa, or millet, but use 1/3 cup water. Add extra water for a creamier texture.

A purée of possibilities

The purées menu opens to expansion at this age. As your baby allows purées of single ingredients to pass Go in the four- to six-months stage, you may start offering combo purées of those foods. Thin purées with extra water if necessary.

Applesauce pumpkin pudding
MAKES 4 SERVINGS

- ¾ cup organic canned pumpkin
- 2 tablespoons organic unsweetened applesauce
- ¼ cup silken tofu (if baby is seven to eight months old)

Whisk ingredients to blend and serve. *(See photo on opposite page.)*

Broccoli-pumpkin purée
MAKES 3–4 OUNCES

- ½ cup fresh organic broccoli florets
- ¼ cup canned organic pumpkin

Lightly steam broccoli in microwave or on stove until soft and bright green. Purée with food processor or food mill. Stir in pumpkin.

Super green purée
MAKES 3–4 OUNCES

- ½ cup frozen organic peas
- 1 cup fresh organic chopped spinach
- ½ cup fresh organic broccoli florets

Steam veggies together over stove or in microwave. Purée with food processor or food mill.

Stewed apricot purée
MAKES 2 SERVINGS

- ¼ cup dried apricots
- ½ cup boiling water

This purée may help constipated babies!

Place apricots in small bowl. Add boiling water. Soak until soft. Pass through baby-food grinder or food processor. Add leftover apricot water to thin purée.

Applesauce pumpkin pudding

Creamy lentil, spinach, potato purée   MAKES 4 CUPS

- 1 medium potato
- 1 cup red lentils
- 2½ cups water
- 1 cup low-sodium chicken broth
- 2 cups fresh spinach leaves
- 1 teaspoon salt

Bake potato in microwave or oven. Meanwhile, place lentils and water in saucepan. Bring water to boil, then reduce heat and simmer lentils until liquid is absorbed, stirring occasionally about 10 to 15 minutes. Add chicken broth and spinach, stir, and simmer for 5 to 10 minutes until spinach is cooked. Stir in salt. Remove from heat. Peel baked potato. Cut potato into chunks and add to lentil mixture. Transfer mixture to food processor or blender and purée until smooth. This purée has a soup consistency and tastes like a pea soup. Add some of your favorite spices and serve for the family too! Purée may need extra water or broth upon reheating to thin to desired consistency.

Banana peach purée   MAKES 12 OUNCES

- 2 medium-size organic peaches
- 1 ripe banana

Peel peaches and slice in half, removing pits. Purée with banana in a blender or food processor.

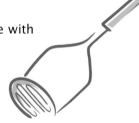

Magnificent mashes

Mashes are a little thicker and offer more texture than purées. If it seems that your baby is managing your purée like a professional, it is probably time to advance to the mash-stage foods. Moms tell me that the avocado mishmash is an all-time favorite.

The montage of mashes below includes fruits, vegetables, and beans that you may serve in single-ingredient dishes or in combination once you know that your baby does not have any allergy or sensitivity to them. Make sure to remove all skins, peels, and seeds from any food to be mashed, and cook vegetables and beans until they are soft.

The mash montage

Fruit mashes (remove skins, peels, and seeds)

Apricots, avocados, bananas, applesauce, cantaloupe, nectarines, pears, peaches, watermelon, plums, and kiwi (kiwi may trigger allergic sensitivities in some babies).

Vegetable mashes (cook veggies until they are soft and remove skins and seeds)

Yellow squash, zucchini, asparagus, broccoli, winter squash, sweet potatoes, yams, potatoes, pumpkin, carrots, green beans, peas, broccoli.

Bean mashes (some babies have trouble digesting beans; wait to serve until your baby is eight months old).

Lentils, black-eyed peas, pinto, garbanzo, lima, black, cannellini, kidney, and soy. Remember that soy may be allergenic, so check for any reaction from your baby when serving soybean mashes.

Chef's suggestions

Frozen or natural-packed organic, canned fruits, veggies, and beans make life easy for the chef! Some markets also offer vacuum-sealed precooked beans and grains. Remove any noticeable skin fibers left in your mash! For easy mashing, pass through baby-food grinder, food mill, or food processor.

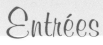

Quick carrot-potato whip

MAKES 8–12 SERVINGS

- 1 pound organic carrots, scrubbed and diced
- 1 medium organic russet potato, peeled and diced
- 1 cup crustless, fresh, wheat-free bread cubes
- 2 tablespoons extra-virgin olive oil
- 2 tablespoons vegetable or chicken broth

Submerge carrots and potato in water and boil or microwave until tender. Drain. Transfer to food processor; purée with bread, oil, and broth. Serve alone or spread on thin slices of crustless, soft bread!

Avocado mishmash

MAKES 4 SERVINGS

- 1 ripe avocado
- ½ cup silken tofu
- 1 ripe banana (if baby is seven to eight months old)

Mash ingredients together and serve! This recipe is a great source of "healthy" fat and a favorite of our clientele. Add some cooked brown rice for a full meal in a mash! *(See photo on opposite page.)*

Egg and edamame mash

MAKES 12 SERVINGS

- 6 hard-boiled egg yolks
- 1 cup cooked edamame
- ¼ cup + 1 tablespoon plain whole-fat yogurt
- 1 tablespoon sweet mustard (brand without honey)

Blend ingredients in a food processor and serve.

Avoid this dish for babies who have soy allergies.

Avocado mishmash

Creamy butternut comfort soup

MAKES 8–10 SERVINGS

- 1 medium butternut squash, halved lengthwise and seeded (approximately 2 cups cooked pulp)
- 2 tablespoons olive oil
- 1 medium sweet onion, chopped
- ¼ teaspoon nutmeg
- ¼ teaspoon cinnamon
- 2 bay leaves
- 1 cup vegetable broth
- 1 medium carrot, coarsely chopped
- 2 celery stalks, chopped
- 1 cup plain, whole-fat soy milk

Poke holes in squash skin and place halves cut-side down to bake or microwave until soft. Bake at 350° for one hour or microwave on vegetable setting. Allow to cool, scoop out pulp into a food processor, and set aside. While squash is cooling, heat oil and sauté chopped onion with spices and bay leaves until onion is soft and translucent. Add carrot and celery with broth and simmer covered until tender (about 10 minutes). Add vegetable mixture (remove bay leaves) to squash in food processor, pour in soy milk, and purée until soup is thick and creamy.

Maize y Manzana mush

MAKES 6 SERVINGS

- 2½ cups water
- ½ cup enriched cornmeal (you may use polenta cornmeal)
- ⅛ teaspoon salt
- 3½ tablespoons unsweetened applesauce
- 3 tablespoons evaporated milk or soy milk

For babies seven months and older

Bring water to a boil. Mix in cornmeal and stir until thickened, approximately 15 minutes. Using hand blender, blend in salt, applesauce, and milk. You may adjust the thickness and taste with additional applesauce and milk. Serve warm. The whole family will enjoy this recipe as hot cereal in the morning or as a side dish at dinner.

Optional: Mix in 1 teaspoon maple syrup per serving for a morning treat.

Not for babies who have corn or cow's milk allergies.

Quinoa and lentil banana pudding   MAKES 16 SERVINGS

- 2½ cups water
- ¾ cup quinoa
- ¼ cup red lentils
- 1 ripe banana
- 1 cup milk or soy milk
- ½ teaspoon vanilla
- 1 teaspoon cinnamon

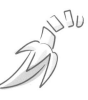

Rinse quinoa. In a medium saucepan, combine water, lentils and quinoa. Bring to a boil, reduce heat and simmer for 15 minutes, stirring occasionally until liquid is absorbed. While the quinoa simmers, in a separate bowl blend together banana, milk, vanilla and cinnamon. Add banana mixture to quinoa and continue to cook, stirring until thick and creamy, approximately 10 more minutes. Remove from heat and cool, and serve.

Treats for teethers

Teething ages are highly individual, and you will be the best judge of when your baby is able to eat textured foods and is ready to order from this teething treat menu. These are great finger foods, too! Beware of choking with any of these foods.

Try these when your baby is ready:

Dry, unsweetened cereals

Zwieback toast, teething crackers, or teething biscuits

Toast corners: Cut the corners off your toast, remove the crust, and serve. Spread with veggie or fruit purées if your baby has not shown an allergic reaction.

Mini-bagel freezes: Thinly slice and freeze a plain mini-bagel, and let your baby gum away!

Frozen peach slivers: Offer your baby a slice of frozen, peeled, fresh, unsweetened canned, or pre-packaged frozen peaches. Cold is soothing to teething babies.

Crunchy crostini: Thinly slice, remove crust, and toast any non-wheat, coarse-textured bread such as ciabatta or rustic varieties.

Finally finger foods

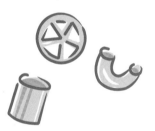

My mom tells me that my favorite game in the finger-food stage was the "uh-oh" game, meaning I would drop foods on the floor and wait for mom to come pick them up, only to "accidentally" throw them on the floor again. If you do not have a dog, finger foods can be a bit messy, but they do allow you freedom in the kitchen to accomplish something besides spoon-feeding your baby. Plastic floor mats can be helpful to manage the occasional and inevitable mess. Some signs that indicate when your baby is ready for finger foods are reaching and grasping for objects, finger dexterity, and bringing the hand to the mouth and teeth! (See Treats for Teethers, p. 75.)

The Chef recommends these finger-food selections:

Fruit: Chopped, skinned pear, apple, peach, apricot, kiwi*, and sliced banana

Vegetables: Chopped, cooked green beans, carrots, broccoli, peas, zucchini, yellow squash, cauliflower, winter squash, potatoes, spinach, and chard

Cooked beans: Garbanzo, lima, pinto, black beans, edamame* (soybeans), lentils, and black-eyed peas

Breads, pastas, rice: Soft, crustless, wheat-free bread, plain muffins, bagels, rolls, cooked wheat-free pastas, and rice varieties (brown, basmati, white) (see Second Servings, Seven- to Eight-Month-Old Diners, p. 64, for additional selections).

* Not for babies allergic to soy.

Country buttermilk oat biscuits
MAKES 4 BISCUITS

- ¼ cup regular or ground oats
- ¼ teaspoon baking soda
- 1½ tablespoons butter or stick margarine (trans-fat free)
- ½ cup unbleached flour
- Pinch of salt
- ¾ teaspoon baking powder
- 1 teaspoon brown sugar
- ⅓ cup buttermilk

Preheat oven to 400°F. Combine dry ingredients. Cut in butter until mixture is a coarse meal. Stir in buttermilk until dough is moist. Sprinkle 1–2 tablespoons flour over cutting board. Knead dough 10 times. Roll into ½-inch thickness and cut into quarters. Place on sprayed cooking sheet. Bake 10 minutes or until lightly browned. Cool and serve in baby-bite pieces!

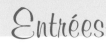

Seashell pasta

MAKES 4 SERVINGS

- 1 cup shell wheat-free pasta
- ½ cup frozen, chopped mixed veggies
- 1 tablespoon olive oil
- ¼ teaspoon salt

Cook pasta as directed on package, drain, and set aside. Steam or microwave veggies. Drain, mix into pasta, toss with olive oil, and serve. Rice or quinoa pastas are good examples of wheat-free alternatives. See Shopping Simplicity, p. 125. *(See photo on opposite page.)*

Pick up soup

MAKES APPROXIMATELY 3 SERVINGS

- 1 can organic, low-sodium, chunky vegetable soup

Drain all liquid, warm slightly, and serve. Seven- to eight-month-old babies may try chicken and vegetable varieties.

Maple parsnip scramble

MAKES 4 SERVINGS

- 2 parsnips, peeled and sliced ¼ inch thick
- 1½ tablespoons canola oil
- 1 tablespoon maple syrup
- Dash of salt and cinnamon

Sauté parsnips in oil over medium heat until soft and golden, approximately 10 minutes. Sprinkle with salt and cinnamon. Remove from heat and stir in maple syrup.

Cool and serve.

Seashell pasta

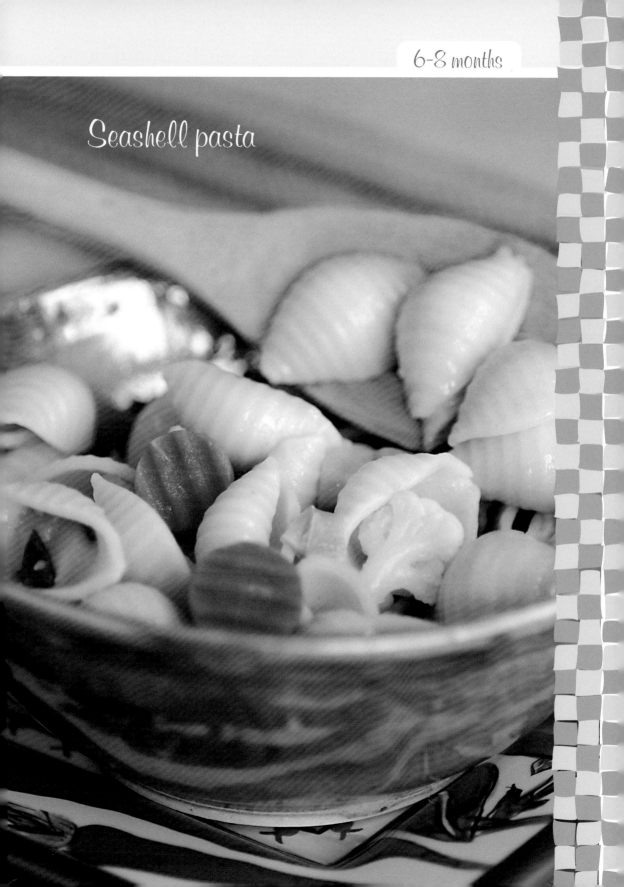

Rainbow roasted veggies

- 1 carrot
- 1 butternut or acorn squash
- 1 yam or sweet potato*
- 2–3 tablespoons olive oil
- 1 zucchini

Preheat oven to 425°. Coat baking sheet with nonstick spray or 1 tablespoon olive oil. Peel carrot, potato, and yam. Slice all veggies into ¼-inch-thick slices. Remove seeds from butternut or acorn squash. Toss veggie slices in olive oil to coat. Place all but zucchini on baking sheet in a single layer. Bake 15–20 minutes on each side or until golden and soft. Add zucchini for last 15 minutes. Cool and cut into bite-size pieces. *(See photo on opposite page.)*

*Sweet potatoes and yams contain more nutrients than white potatoes and do not elevate blood sugar as rapidly.

Open-face finger sandwiches with turkey-asparagus paté
MAKES APPROXIMATELY 4 SANDWICHES

- 1 piece soft, thin, wheat-free sandwich bread
- 2 tablespoons cooked brown short-grain rice
- 2 tablespoons cooked frozen or fresh asparagus tips
- ⅓ cup cooked turkey meat*
- 2 tablespoons veggie broth or cooking water from veggies

Remove crust from bread. Pass turkey, rice, and asparagus through baby-food grinder, food mill, or food processor. Blend with broth. Spread in thin layer onto bread and cut into small 1-inch squares for baby bites. You may substitute any frozen or fresh cooked veggies you have available.

*Leave out the meat for babies less than seven months old.

Rainbow roasted veggies

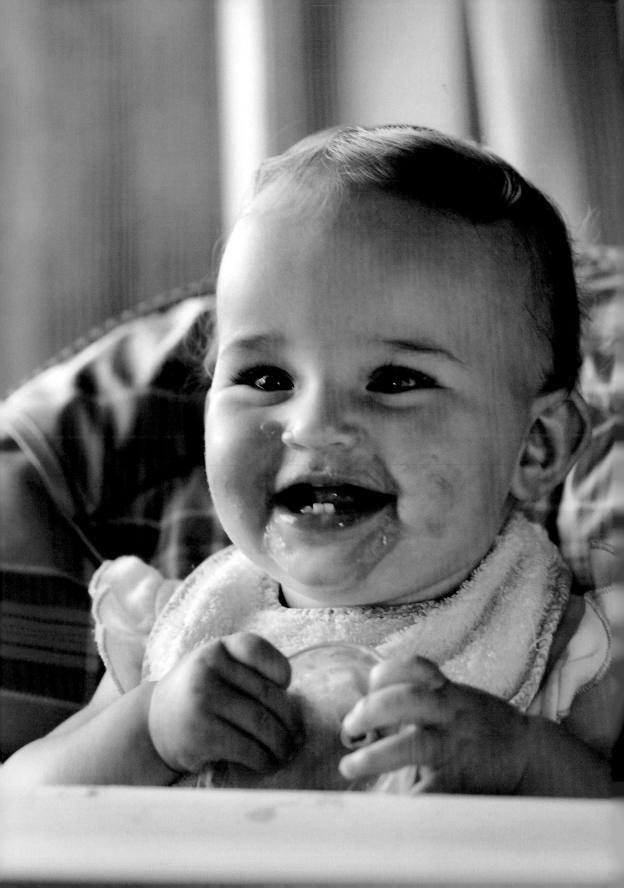

Entrées

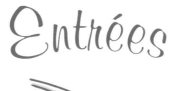

Eight to twelve months

Babies change so quickly it is hard to keep up! Their emerging personalities are a joy to behold, they are sleeping with fewer awakenings in the night, they notice more and more of their surroundings, and they still like green veggies (just wait until the toddler years . . .). As that first birthday approaches, purées and mashes evolve into soft, more textured meals for your developing baby to devour.

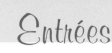

Nutrient needs

This chart is identical to the six to eight months chart except for one new note: Your baby's birth weight is expected to triple by twelve months! Flex those biceps; you may become a threat to the current world arm-wrestling champion!

Calorie, protein, and fat intake for eight to twelve months			
Pounds	Calories/Day	Protein(g)/Day	Fat(g)/Day
15	670	11	31
17	760	13	35
19	850	14	39
21	940	16	44
23	1,030	17	48
25	1,110	19	52
27	1,200	20	56
30	1,340	23	62

Premature or other special-needs babies may have supplemental requirements. Check with your health care provider.

Serving suggestions

Check out the fat!

Fat equals almost half a day's calories!
1 gram = 9 calories

Adjusting to solid foods is important for your baby's coordination and acceptance of new culinary appearances, textures, and tastes. You have already established the basics of feeding some foods. As your baby matures, keep building those eating skills with the following tips.

- Offer thicker (mashed) foods and more chopped or sliced table foods.
- Offer a wider variety of meats or meat substitutes.
- Offer more finger foods as your baby's hand coordination improves.
- Adjust textured foods according to dental maturity. Anything can be puréed!
- Keep encouraging the sippy cup.
- Keep encouraging self-feeding; this means freedom for you, too!
- Remember the "Sweeter Later" rule: Bitter foods may be more popular if they come before sweeter selections!
- Make extra batches of your special recipes and staple foods like rice or purées to refrigerate or freeze for later days.

More on the menu

This is about that time when your baby accepts and is able to digest a variety of foods, but you are stuck in a rut as to what new dishes to try. The Combo Cuisine section will help inspire your creativity to serve a well-balanced, delicious dish with whatever you may have in the freezer, pantry, or refrigerator. Finger-food frenzy is for the growing crowd of babies out there who are practicing to get five out of five bites in their mouths all by themselves. Pictures please! If you have favorite candid camera shots of your baby's colorful attempt to maneuver food from plate to mouth, send them to me at bbb@babybistrobrands.com. I love to post pictures on the Bistro Babies page.

If you are more of a shopper than chef, feel free to flip to Appendix 2, p. 125, for some brand suggestions.

Combo cuisine

Think outside the box in blending foods from different groups in Baby's Grand Buffet, or go for one of the tried and true recipes that follow. Thin any combo with one to two tablespoons of broth, cooking water, olive or canola oil, breast milk, formula, or rice cereal for a creamy texture.

All meals should be served with breast milk, iron-fortified formula, or iron-fortified soy formula for vegan clientele.

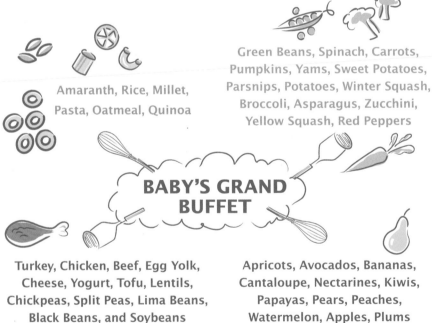

Amaranth, Rice, Millet, Pasta, Oatmeal, Quinoa

Green Beans, Spinach, Carrots, Pumpkins, Yams, Sweet Potatoes, Parsnips, Potatoes, Winter Squash, Broccoli, Asparagus, Zucchini, Yellow Squash, Red Peppers

BABY'S GRAND BUFFET

Turkey, Chicken, Beef, Egg Yolk, Cheese, Yogurt, Tofu, Lentils, Chickpeas, Split Peas, Lima Beans, Black Beans, and Soybeans

Apricots, Avocados, Bananas, Cantaloupe, Nectarines, Kiwis, Papayas, Pears, Peaches, Watermelon, Apples, Plums

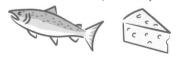
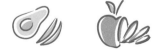

Sweet and natural carrot cake muffins

MAKES 12 REGULAR OR
4 DOZEN MINI-MUFFINS

- 1¾ cups unbleached flour (for babies older than 12 months, substitute ¾ cup whole wheat flour for ¾ cup white flour)
- 1 teaspoon nutmeg
- ½ teaspoon baking soda
- 2 teaspoons baking powder
- Pinch of salt
- 1 teaspoon cinnamon
- 1 red or Gala apple, peeled, cored, and grated
- 1 large carrot, peeled and grated
- 1 cup buttermilk
- 1 large egg, beaten
- ½ cup mashed, ripe bananas (about 2 small bananas)
- 4 tablespoons dark brown sugar

Preheat the oven to 350°. Line a muffin pan with papers or lightly spray with oil.

Mix the dry ingredients except sugar in a medium bowl. In a small bowl, combine the apple and carrot. Stir in the buttermilk, egg, banana, and sugar. Stir in the dry ingredients, avoiding overmixing. Spoon into the muffin pan. Bake 20 minutes for regular muffins or 10 minutes for mini-muffins.

Chef's secret

No peeling needed for apples if you cut them into quarters, then core and grate them against a cheese grater with the peel side out. The peel will not grate and the apple will!

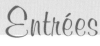

Healthy chicken-apple nuggets

MAKES 20 NUGGETS

- 1 red or Gala apple, peeled, cored, and grated
- ½ cup chopped red onion
- 3–4 tablespoons minced fresh parsley
- 2 boneless, skinless chicken breasts cut into chunks (about 2 cups) for pan-browning
- ¾ cup raw oatmeal
- 1 tablespoon low-sodium chicken broth
- 1 tablespoon canola oil
- Unbleached flour, for coating

Wrap the grated apple in paper towel and squeeze out the excess juice (see Chef's Secret on page 87 for tips on apple grating). Combine the chicken, apple, onion, oats, broth, and parsley in a food processor. Mix well. Spread about 2 tablespoons of flour on a plate.

Hand-form rounded spoonfuls of the chicken mixture to create small, round balls and roll them in the flour. Heat the oil in a nonstick skillet over medium heat. Pan-brown the chicken nuggets until golden and cooked through. Drain on paper towel. Delicious hot, cold or added to soups and sauces! Make sure you carefully wash your hands, cutting board and utensils after handling raw chicken. *(See photo on opposite page.)*

Spinach cheese squares

MAKES 8 SERVINGS

- 2 cups cooked, chopped spinach
- 1 cup wheat-free bread crumbs
- 1½ cups grated cheddar or jack cheese
- 1 tablespoon extra-virgin olive oil

Mix all the ingredients. Press into a greased 8" x 8" x 2" baking dish. Bake at 350° for 45 minutes. Cut into squares and serve!

Healthy chicken-apple nuggets

Entrées

Salmon potato cakes*

MAKES 8 SERVINGS

- 2 cups canned, drained salmon (haddock, cod, or flounder is OK, too)
- 2 cups cooked diced or mashed potatoes
- 1–2 egg yolks
- Wheat-free bread crumbs

*Not for families with a history of egg or fish allergies.

Mix the salmon, potatoes, and egg yolks and shape into small cakes. Dip in bread crumbs. Slowly sauté in canola oil, olive oil, or ghee on both sides until browned. *(See photo on opposite page.)*

Simple chicken and shells soup

MAKES 4–6 SERVINGS

- 3 cups low-sodium chicken broth
- 1 cup dried, wheat-free elbow macaroni or shell pasta
- 1 cup frozen mixed vegetables
- 1¾ cups cooked chopped chicken (approximately 3 cooked chicken breasts)
- 2 teaspoons Italian seasoning
- 1 bay leaf

In medium saucepan, bring the broth to a simmer. Add the pasta and cook for 5 minutes. Add the vegetables, chicken, and seasonings. Cook for 10 minutes or until the pasta is soft and the veggies are heated through. Serve with soft bread bits.

Vegan variation: Substitute extra-firm tofu and vegetable broth for the chicken and chicken broth.

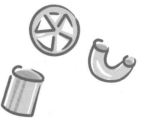

Salmon potato cakes

Creamy sweet potato-pumpkin soup

MAKES 6 SERVINGS

- 1 tablespoon olive oil
- ¾ cup chopped yellow onion
- 1 garlic clove, minced
- ¼ teaspoon nutmeg
- 1 teaspoon ginger
- ½ teaspoon curry powder
- ¼ teaspoon cumin
- ¼ teaspoon cinnamon
- 2 cups peeled, cubed sweet potato
- 2 cups low-sodium chicken broth
- 1½ cups water
- 1 15-ounce can of pumpkin
- 1 cup milk
- 3 tablespoons plain yogurt

Choose organic brands if possible. Vegans may substitute soy milk, soy yogurt, and veggie broth. Heat the olive oil in a large pot over medium-high heat. Add the onion and sauté until it's clear and tender. Stir in the spices and garlic and cook 1 to 2 minutes. Add the sweet potato, broth, water, and pumpkin. Bring to a boil. Reduce heat and simmer for 20 minutes or until the sweet potato is soft. Remove from heat and stir in the milk. Transfer to a food processor and purée. Serve warm with a dollop of plain yogurt. *(See photo on opposite page.)*

Spinach special

MAKES 8 SERVINGS

- 10 ounces fresh or frozen cooked, chopped spinach
- ½ pound (8 ounces) ground turkey, tofu, or tempeh
- 2 eggs
- 1–2 tablespoons olive or canola oil

Stir-fry meat or meat substitute with oil in a skillet. Scramble in eggs; add spinach over low heat. Top with grated cheese or cheese alternative.

Creamy sweet potato-pumpkin soup

Delicious golden dal

MAKES 16 OUNCES

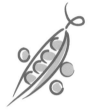

- 1 cup red lentils
- ¾ cup chopped yellow, sweet onion
- ½ cup diced, peeled sweet potato
- ½ cup frozen peas
- ½ cup peeled carrot, sliced ¼ inch thick
- 1 cup chopped, fresh spinach (optional)
- ¼ teaspoon cumin
- ½ teaspoon cinnamon
- ½ teaspoon ginger
- ½ teaspoon salt
- ½ teaspoon curry powder

Place the lentils, onion, and sweet potato in a medium-size pot with 2 ½ cups of water and salt. Bring to a boil. Reduce heat and simmer uncovered for 20 minutes, stirring often. Add the peas, carrots, and spinach. Stir and simmer 10 more minutes. Mix in the spices. Simmer until the extra liquid is gone and the lentils are blended to a creamy texture. Purée according to dentition.

Cowboy black bean-rice bake

MAKES 12–16 SERVINGS

- 1½ cups cooked short-grain brown rice
- ½ cup plain yogurt
- ⅔ cup cooked black beans
- 1 zucchini, thinly sliced (Hint: Use the slicer side of your cheese grater!)
- ¾ cup grated cheddar cheese

Preheat the oven to 350°. Lightly spray an 8" square baking dish. Mix rice, beans, and yogurt in a small bowl. Spread mixture into the bottom of a baking dish. Arrange a single layer of squash slices over the rice mix. Sprinkle cheese evenly over the squash. Bake for 25 to 30 minutes. Cool and serve.

Finger-food frenzy

Here are more easy and healthy finger-food recipes that can feed the rest of the family, too. Serve your baby single servings cut into baby bite-sized pieces. Some parents say that the sweet potato-molasses-spinach muffins are the only way their baby will eat spinach and tried to convince me to go into the muffin business!

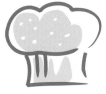

Favorite fake fries   **MAKES 3 TO 4 SERVINGS**

- 2 parsnips peeled, cut in half, and then quartered lengthwise to resemble fries
- 1 tablespoon olive or canola oil
- Sprinkle of salt and pepper

Preheat the oven to 425°. Toss the parsnips in the oil. Place in a single layer on an oiled or foil-covered baking sheet. Sprinkle with salt and pepper. Bake for 20 minutes, 10 minutes on each side. Serve with a little ketchup. Try fake frying sweet potatoes, too!

Tofu scramble   **MAKES 4 SERVINGS**

- 8 ounces firm tofu
- 1 cup hot water
- 1 tablespoon brown rice syrup or maple syrup

Crumble the tofu into a large, dry skillet. Whisk the water and syrup. Stir into the skillet and simmer over high heat. When bubbling, lower the heat to medium, stirring occasionally until the liquid is gone or the tofu is moist and soft (15 to 20 minutes).

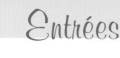

Broccoli trees

MAKES 4 SERVINGS

- 2 cups chopped fresh or frozen, thawed broccoli

Steam or microwave the broccoli until soft. Cool and serve! Try topping with 1 tablespoon grated cheese or baby's other favorite flavor if plain broccoli does not pass inspection! *(See photo on opposite page.)*

Evan's oatmeal bars

MAKES 4 TO 6 SERVINGS

- 1 cup raw oatmeal
- ⅔ cup skinned, diced fruit (apple, apricots, raisins)
- 1¾ cups water
- ¼ teaspoon cinnamon

Preheat the oven to 325°. Mix the ingredients in a shallow glass baking dish. Microwave to cook the oatmeal (3 to 4 minutes on high power). Transfer to the oven and bake for 20 to 25 minutes until lightly golden and the liquid is absorbed. Cut into pieces and serve!

Quesadilla triangles

MAKES 8 SERVINGS

- 2 flour tortillas
- ¾ cup grated jack or cheddar cheese
- ½ cup finely chopped or grated veggie (broccoli, carrot, red bell pepper, squash)
- 2 tablespoons mashed pinto beans or 100 percent organic refried beans (optional)

If using mashed beans, spread them onto one flour tortilla and sprinkle the chopped veggies on top. Place the tortilla in a skillet over medium heat. Cover evenly with the grated cheese and top with the second tortilla. Cook on both sides until the cheese is melted. Cut into small triangles and serve!

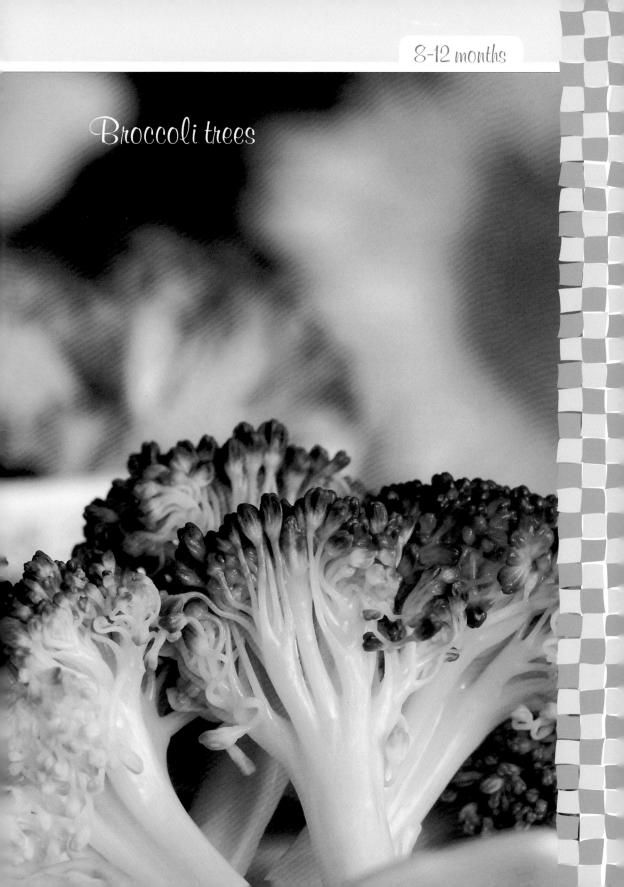

Broccoli trees

Toasted cheese bread

MAKES 4 TO 8 SERVINGS

- 2 slices of any wheat-free bread, crusts removed
- 2 thin slices of jack or cheddar cheese

Preheat the oven to 350°. Top bread with the cheese slices and toast in the oven until the cheese is melted. Serve in bite-size pieces.

Adam's eggless bananawama muffins

MAKES 4 DOZEN MINI-MUFFINS

- 2 ripe (1 cup) mashed bananas
- ¼ cup canola oil
- ¾ cup plain whole-fat yogurt
- ¾ cup unsweetened apricot applesauce (or baby-food version)
- 1 teaspoon vanilla
- 1 cup baby rolled oats
- 2 cups unbleached flour
- ⅓ cup brown sugar
- 1 teaspoon nutmeg
- ½ teaspoon cinnamon
- 1½ teaspoons baking powder
- 1 teaspoon baking soda

Preheat the oven to 375°. Mix the wet ingredients in a large bowl. Mix the dry ingredients in a small bowl and then add to the wet ingredients. Combine. Spoon into lined or sprayed mini-muffin tins. Bake for 10 to 12 minutes. If using regular muffin tins, bake for 20 minutes.

Freeze extras!

Broccolicious cheesy buttermilk muffins

MAKES 12 REGULAR MUFFINS

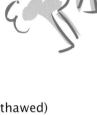

- 1 cup buttermilk
- 2 tablespoons canola oil
- 1 cup unsweetened applesauce or 6 ounces of silken tofu, beat smooth
- 1½ tablespoons maple syrup
- 1¾ cups unbleached flour
- ¼ teaspoon salt
- 2 teaspoons baking powder
- 1 cup grated cheddar cheese
- ½ cup finely chopped broccoli, fresh or frozen (thawed)

Preheat the oven to 400°. Mix the wet ingredients in a medium-size bowl. Stir in the dry ingredients. Add the cheese and broccoli. Spoon the mixture into sprayed or lined regular muffin tins. Bake for 20 to 25 minutes.

Yogurt cheese on pita pieces

MAKES 6 SERVINGS

- 1 cup Greek yogurt (whole-fat)
- 1 plain, soft pita bread

Line a small sieve with a dampened paper towel and set over a bowl or cup so that the bottom of the sieve is not touching the base of its container. Spoon the yogurt into the sieve. Place in the refrigerator for 3 hours. The yogurt will be drained of extra liquid and delicious cheese will be left! Spread onto small, bite-sized pita pieces. You may also mix the cheese into rice, cereals, pasta, or vegetables to add a creamy texture.

If you can't find Greek yogurt, you may use regular whole-fat plain yogurt. Just increase draining time in the fridge to overnight.

Sweet potato-molasses-spinach muffins

MAKES 4 DOZEN MINI-MUFFINS

- 1 cup mashed, cooked sweet potato (microwaved, not boiled)
- ¼ cup chopped organic raisins
- 1 cup chopped, fresh spinach
- 2 eggs
- ½ cup buttermilk
- ⅓ cup molasses
- ¼ cup canola oil
- 1¾ cup unbleached flour
- ½ cup light brown sugar
- 1 teaspoon cinnamon
- ⅓ teaspoon ginger
- 1 teaspoon baking soda
- 1 teaspoon baking powder
- ¼ teaspoon salt

Preheat the oven to 375°. Line mini-muffin tins. Mix the raisins, sweet potatoes, spinach, and wet ingredients in a bowl until smooth, and mix the dry ingredients in another bowl. Combine the two and mix until blended. Spoon the batter into muffin tins and bake on the middle shelf until lightly browned (about 10 minutes for mini-muffins). Delicious and loaded with vitamin A and iron! *(See photo on opposite page.)*

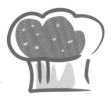

Sweet potato-
molasses-spinach
muffins

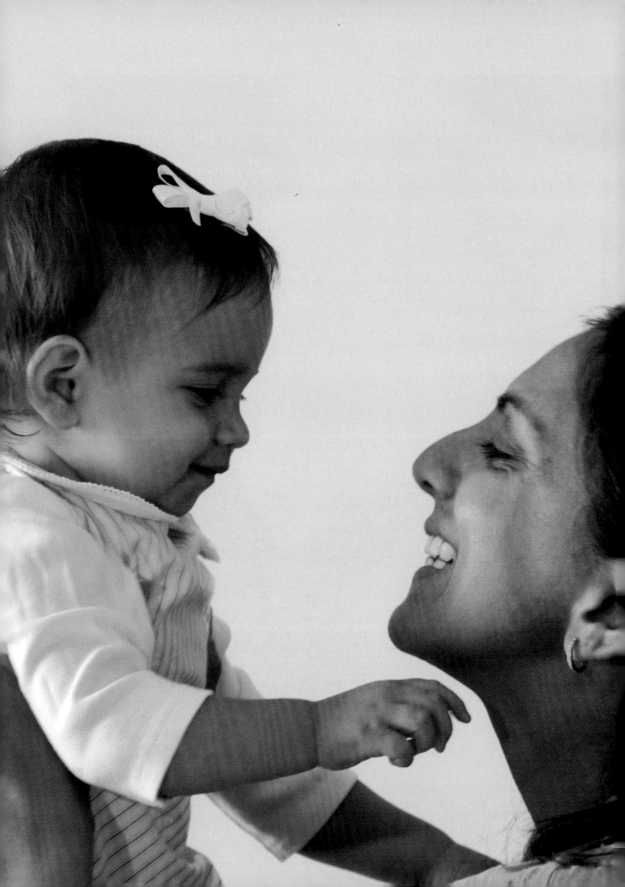

À la Carte

Supplements for babies and pregnant or breast-feeding moms

À la Carte is all about getting you "in the know" about the stand-out nutrients that are so important for your and your baby's health. The answers to questions you have, and those you don't even know to ask about supplements, like "what, when, why, and how much?" are all presented here for you to order up as needed.

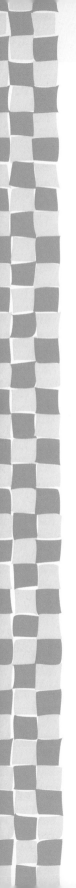

Á la Carte

For the baby

You are juggling so much with a new baby you can barely keep your head on straight. In between the diaper cleaning, naps, feedings, doctor appointments, postpartum group meetings, and trying to get back to a fraction of work and friend life before baby, making sure your baby is getting enough of certain nutrients is just beyond imagination. Isn't breast-feeding enough?

Breast-feeding is fabulous, but modern living has left a few nutrients in need of a boost in your baby's diet from supplemental sources. In addition, babies may or may not need certain supplements depending on their unique situation, such as being raised on a vegan diet.

Vitamin D

Vitamin D supports proper bone growth and density, muscle strength, and immune activity and may help to ward off colon cancer and type 1 diabetes. We make our own vitamin D with adequate sun exposure. Research increasingly indicates, however, that unless you live close to the equator, most of us do not have appropriate blood levels of vitamin D. Cold, dark climates, sunscreens, and dark skin decrease your ability to produce vitamin D. The American Academy of Pediatrics recommends that all nursing mothers supplement their babies with vitamin D for the duration of breast-feeding. Food sources of vitamin D are fatty fish and fortified beverages and yogurts. Vitamin drops are available over the counter or by prescription. Discuss options with your health care provider.

From birth to twelve months, the recommended amount babies need is 400 international units (IUs) per day. Breast milk contains about 22 to 25 IUs per liter.

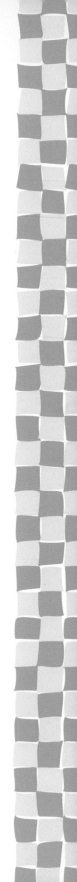

> **Bistro Bests**
>
> **NutriStart Multivitamin Powder** by Rainbow Light (Santa Cruz, California) Serve one-half packet per day for six- to twelve-month-olds; includes 200 IUs of vitamin D.

DHA

DHA (docosahexanoic acid) is an omega-3 fatty acid vital to brain and visual development. In fact, it is the most abundant fatty acid in the brain! DHA is a natural ingredient in breast milk. If you do not breast-feed, make sure that your formula contains DHA, or you may add a DHA supplement to your formula, yogurt, or purées. Research indicates that children whose diets were supplemented with DHA in infancy show improved visual acuity and IQ scores, as well as lower blood pressure. Flavored liquid DHA is available for weaned babies and young children.

From birth to twelve months, include about 100 milligrans per day in your baby's diet.

> **Bistro Bests**
>
> **Carlson for Kids Very Finest Fish Oil** (Arlington Heights, Illinois). Lemon-flavored, naturally sweetened; one-fourth teaspoon contains 125 milligrams of DHA.

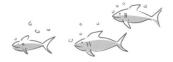

Á la Carte

Vitamin K

Babies should receive a vitamin K injection at birth. This treatment is necessary to prevent hemorrhagic disease of the newborn.
From birth to six months, the adequate intake of two micrograms (µg) per day is met by the injection at birth and the amount in breast milk or formula. After six months, vitamin K is sufficiently supplied from formula, breast milk, and supplemental weaning foods. The recommended amount is 2.5 µg/day.

Probiotics (i.e. L. Bifidobacteria, L. acidophilus, L. bulgaricus, L. rhamnosus, L. thermophilus)

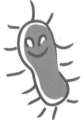

Probiotics, meaning "pro-life," are the friendly bacteria living in our intestines. Studies link probiotics with many benefits, such as limiting lactose intolerance, helping to prevent symptoms of colic and food allergy reactions, in at-risk infants, synthesizing nutrients, increasing nutrient absorption, and boosting the immune system by protecting against infectious bacteria.

Breast milk contains growth factors that help these bacteria grow in your baby's intestines. You may want to consider infant probiotics if you formula-feed using a brand that does not contain natural bacterial cultures or if your baby is susceptible to infections or diarrhea.

Probiotics supplements:

- **Baby's Jarro-Dophilus, Jarrow Formulas** (Canada)
- **Ultra Bifidus, DF, Metagenics** (San Clemente, California)
- **Nature's Way Primadophilus for Children or Kids** (Springville, Utah)

- **Nutrition Now Rhino FOS and Acidophilus** (Vancouver, Washington)

Find these powder supplements in the refrigerated or vitamin section of health food stores. Mix the specified serving size with the baby food or beverage.

Refrigerated brands will keep for three to six weeks in your refrigerator after opening, and shelf-stable brands will save for twelve months. Check www.consumerlab.com for reviews on specific brands. Please note: Probiotics are not yet FDA approved. Consult your health care provider first if you're considering them for your baby.

Bistro Bests Find probiotics in whole fat yogurts for infants older than seven months. Be a CLR (Compulsive Label Reader) for the "Live Active Culture" seal.

Iron

Red blood cells use iron to transport oxygen in our blood, which is necessary for normal cognitive and physical development. Iron deficiency and iron-deficiency anemia are associated with decreased learning, attention span, and motor and behavioral functioning, and can be irreversible. Formula-fed infants should receive only iron-fortified formula (4 to 12 milligrams per liter). There is no proof that the amount of iron in formulas causes constipation or colic. By six months of age, breast-fed babies need iron from solid weaning foods in addition to the iron supplied in breast milk.

Á la Carte

Babies seven to twelve months of age need 11 milligrams of iron per day. Do not exceed 15 milligrams per day.

Incredible iron sources

> 2 ounces fortified cereal = 5 milligrams
> 1 tablespoon blackstrap molasses = 5 milligrams
> 2 ounces cooked beans = 1.5 milligams
> 2 ounces cooked fresh spinach = 1.5 milligrams
> 1 ounce beef = 1 milligram
> 2 ounces tofu = 0.9 milligram
> 1 ounce poultry = 0.5 milligram
> 1 ounce fish= 0.3 milligram
> 1 kiwi = 0.3 milligram

Bistro Bests **Iron** from meats, poultry, and fish is more easily absorbed than iron from plant sources. Fruits and vegetables high in vitamin C or vitamin C supplements, and foods rich in protein increase iron absorption.

Fluoride

Fluoride is essential to build strong teeth and bones and helps to prevent dental caries. Babies who are exposed to excessive fluoride while their enamel is forming, however, may be at an increased risk for fluorosis, which appears as stained or pitted tooth enamel.

You may need to give your baby a fluoride supplement if you breast-feed and do not drink fluoridated water or if you formula-feed and use unfluoridated water or tap water that contains less than 0.3 parts per million (ppm) of fluoride.

The area where you live may have water that naturally contains fluoride or your community may have a water fluoridation program. Many states list their water fluoridation status on the Centers for Disease Control and Prevention, My Water's Fluoride web site. Check it out at http://apps.nccd.cdc.gov/MWF/Index.asp and talk to your health care provider or pediatric dentist about your baby's fluoride intake.

The recommended amount of fluoride for babies seven to twelve months of age is 0.5 milligrams per day. If your doctor decides that you should give your baby a supplement, the amount is usually 0.25 milligrams per day in a fluoride drop formulation.

For the vegan baby

Families practicing vegan diets are generally healthy and very nutrition savvy. Raising a vegan baby, however, does require some extra vigilance to include important nutrients that mostly come from the animal kingdom.

Vitamin B12

Vitamin B12 is important for growth and nerve development. B12 is found mainly in animal products, milk, and dairy. If you are a vegan and are breast-feeding exclusively, make sure that vitamin B12 is in your daily vitamin and in your diet. You may also need to give your baby a B12 supplement, and when your baby is ready for solid foods, include B12-fortified cereals and meat alternatives on the menu. Discuss B12 supplements with your health care provider.

Babies need 0.4 µg per day of vitamin B12 from birth to six months and 0.5 µg per day from seven to twelve months of age.

Zinc

Zinc is important for normal growth, development, and immune system defense. Low-birth-weight infants are given zinc in third world countries to help prevent diarrhea caused by infection. Zinc is found in meat, fish, and eggs. Although it is also in whole grains and beans, these foods contain "phytates," which can bind zinc, effectively trapping it and blocking its absorption. Vegan foods that help zinc absorption are yeast-leavened breads and fermented soy products. Weaned babies may need a zinc supplement if their diets lack zinc-rich foods.

Babies ages seven to twelve months need 3 milligrams per day of zinc.

For pregnant and breast-feeding moms

When you are pregnant or breast-feeding, the last thing you may want to do is to remember to take a nutrient supplement, but your body and your growing baby require extra nutrient side orders to keep the mommy and baby train on track.

The Baby Bistro's favorite prenatal vitamins and minerals for pregnant and lactating moms

Hundreds of prenatal supplements are out there to confuse you, so Baby Bistro presents an ideal ingredient list of vitamins and minerals and their recommended amounts to help you choose the best options. Look for the following ingredients on prenatal brand labels. If you are overwhelmed by just glancing at labels, see p. 114 for "Bistro Bests" prenatal brand suggestions.

The Baby Bistro's favorite prenatal vitamins and minerals for pregnant and lactating moms

Vitamin	Form	DRI* (pregnant)	DRI* (lactating)
A	beta-carotene or mixed carotenes	4,620 IUs	7,800 IUs
D	D3 or cholecalciferol	200 IUs	200 IUs
E	d-alpha-tocopherol or mixed tocopherols	15 IUs	19 IUs
K	phylloquinone	90 µg	90 µg
C	ascorbic acid	85 mg	120 mg
	Vitamin C defends against preeclampsia and PROM (premature rupture of the fetal membrane).		
B1	thiamin or thiamin HCL	1.4 mg	1.4 mg
B2	riboflavin	1.4 mg	1.6 mg
B3	niacin, nicotinic acid	18 mg	17 mg
B5	pantothenic acid	6 mg	7 mg
B6	pyridoxine, pyridoxal-5-phosphate	1.9 mg	2.0 mg
Folic Acid	folic acid, folate	600 µg	500 µg
	Folate is very important in preventing neural tube defects.		
B12	methylcobalamin	2.6 µg	2.8 µg
Biotin	biotin, biocytin	30 µg	35 µg
Choline	450 mg	550 mg	
	Choline is essential to brain development.		

*DRI – Dietary Reference Intake

Á la Carte

Mineral	Form	DRI* (pregnant)	DRI* (lactating)
calcium	calcium citrate or malate	1,000 mg	1,000 mg
magnesium	magnesium citrate	350 mg	310 mg
Magnesium is associated with preventing preeclampsia.			
potassium	potassium chloride or aspartate	4,700 mg	5,100 mg
zinc	zinc picolinate, citrate	11 mg	12 mg
Zinc is associated with preventing low birth weight.			
copper	copper sulfate, picolinate	1,000 µg	1,300 µg
iron	ferrous succinate, sulfate, bisglycinate	27 mg	9 mg
selenium	selenomethionine	60 µg	70 µg
Selenium is associated with preventing low birth weight and SIDS.			

*DRI – Dietary Reference Intake

FYI

Beware! If your vitamin A is in the form of retinol or retinyl palmitate, it may accumulate to toxic levels in the body. Ingesting more than 10,000 IUs per day in this form may cause birth defects and liver damage. The Dietary Reference Intake for this form is 2,541 IUs during pregnancy or 4,290 IUs during lactation. Note that in the Baby Bistro prenatal recipe, the suggested amounts are in the safer form, beta carotene, which your body converts to vitamin A.

"Docusate sodium" may also appear on some prenatal ingredient labels. This is a stool softener to counteract constipation caused by some forms of iron. Follow the "WEW" tips below and look for iron in more digestive-friendly formulations, such as ferrous bisglycinate, if you want to avoid docusate sodium.

"WEW" spells relief versus constipation

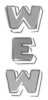

Water: four sixteen-ounce glasses per day

Eat fibrous foods (fruits, veggies, whole grains)

Work out with daily exercise, even if only for a few minutes!

Follow these self-service suggestions for taking your prenatal supplement.

Follow the instructions on the container.

- Take with water or juice. Milk, coffee, and tea decrease absorption.

- Don't take with a high-fiber meal. Fibrous veggies and grains contain "phytates" that can decrease absorption of minerals like iron, zinc, and calcium.

- If your prenatal supplement contains iron, take a separate calcium supplement at a different time, and with a meal. Calcium and iron (in your prenatal vitamin) compete for absorption, and iron wins.

- Foods high in vitamin C, a vitamin C supplement, or high-protein foods like meat, fish, or poultry, help iron absorption.

Á la Carte

Choose your prenatal vitamin from these Bistro Best recommendations:

- **Rainbow Light Prenatal One Multivitamin** (Santa Cruz, California). Yipee! You only have to take one a day! You do need to take an extra calcium supplement (1,000 milligrams per day). This supplement also contains red raspberry and ginger to aid with morning sickness.

- **TwinLab Prenatal Care Multivitamin Caps** (American Fork, Utah). You take two per day, and the iron is in the form of bisglycinate, which is less likely to cause constipation. You do need to take a separate calcium supplement to ensure proper iron absorption.

- **NOW Prenatal Capsules** (Bloomingdale, Illinois). You take four per day. This prenatal also contains the full DRI (Dietary Reference Intake) for calcium and has iron in the form of bisglycinate. Capsules also dissolve and absorb easily.

Prescription prenatals such as OptiNate and Duet DHA are also good choices. These are tablets packaged with DHA capsules.

DHA

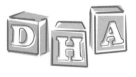

DHA (docosahexaenoic acid) is an omega-3 fatty acid and is the most abundant type of fat in our brains. Associated with enhanced cognitive development and visual acuity in newborns, it is especially needed during the last trimester of pregnancy. Food sources are primarily cold-water fish and fortified eggs. Vegan moms should take DHA during pregnancy and lactation. Studies have linked higher IQs and better vision with infants breast-fed by moms taking a DHA supplement. Women with a history of miscarriage may also benefit.

DHA capsules are either fish oil–based or algae-grown. You may find the algae-grown capsule to be less fishy tasting than the fish-oil brands. The World Health Organization (WHO) Suggests 300 milligrams per day of DHA for pregnant women.

FYI: DHA levels in American women's breast milk are among the lowest in the world! Placing last in the world breast milk DHA competition is not a good thing. This reflects the typical "western diet" and is one more reason to take a DHA supplement.

Choose your DHA supplement from these Bistro Best recommendations:

- **Mead Johnson Expecta LIPIL** (Evansville, Indiana) algae-grown, 200-milligram capsules

- **Source Naturals DHA** (Scotts Valley, California) algae-grown, 100-milligram capsules

- **Nature's Way Neuromins** (Springville, Utah) plant-sourced DHA, 100-milligram capsules

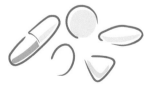

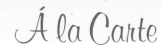

Á la Carte

For pregnant and breast-feeding vegan moms

Because you don't eat meat, make sure that your diet includes alternative sources of iron-rich foods and that your prenatal supplement contains iron. Iron protects against iron-deficiency anemia and is essential to normal growth and development for your baby! Zinc, calcium, and vitamins D, B12, and B6, are also more meat-biased nutrients that vegan moms should maintain in their diet with their prenatal supplement and fortified foods.

Iron-packed eats

Many plant foods contain iron, but some do not provide iron in a way that makes it available for us to absorb. The following foods are rich in iron that is usable by our bodies. These foods are healthy for vegan moms throughout pregnancy, breast-feeding, and beyond!

- **Fruits**
  Oranges, cantaloupe, mangos, guavas, dried fruits

- **Vegetables**
  Beets, broccoli, cabbage, cauliflower, pumpkin, turnips, tomatoes, carrots, potatoes, dark green, leafy vegetables, sea vegetables (nori, arame, hijiki)

- **Other recommendations**
  Corn flour, white flour, iron-fortified cereals, millet, oats, quinoa, Brewer's yeast, unleavened bread, blackstrap molasses, beans

- Remember, vitamin C–rich foods or supplements and protein foods help iron absorption!

Supplement savvy

Supplements are not all created equal; higher cost doesn't necessarily equal better! Look at the label—this is where you'll find the information you need to make good, educated purchases. Take note of the following label highlights to enhance your supplement shopping expertise and to help you refine your search.

Check for:

- **% DRI (Dietary Reference Intake) or DV (Daily Value)/serving**
  This tells you what percentage of the government recommended amount of the nutrient you are going to get from the serving size on the label.

- **Formulation of nutrient**
  The nutrient "formula" is the chemical makeup that the manufacturer has chosen. It follows the name of the nutrient on the label.

- **Binders, fillers, or other additives**
  Capsules can be made without these, but tablets cannot. If you have extreme allergies, you may need a supplement that contains no wheat, corn, milk, yeast, fillers, additives, artificial colors, or flavors.

- **Daily dose**
  It's a pain to take eight capsules for the desired daily dose. Look for more swallowable options.

- **Expiration date**
  Supplements last eighteen to twenty-four months. Throw them out six months after the expiration date. Probiotics last twelve months or less and should be discarded on the expiration date.

- **Container color**
  Opaque or dark color equals better preservation. Supplements generally like places that are dark and cool. Transparent containers allow light and heat to penetrate through, which may alter the chemical integrity of the nutrients.

Supplement science for those inquiring minds

Vitamin formulations are synthetic or natural. Synthetic vitamins have a "dl-" preceding the name. Natural vitamins have a "d-" preceding the name.

Mineral formulations are inorganic salts or organic acids. If the mineral is chelated (bonded) to an amino acid, it is considered to be in its "organic" form. The amino acid should be identified on the label next to the mineral name. The amino acid chelates usually end in an "-ate," like "citrate." Inorganic mineral forms commonly have the mineral followed by an "oxide," except for "carbonate" or "sulfate."

Who cares?

The theory is that the natural, organic forms are more easily absorbed by the body. Another theory is that a vitamin may be better absorbed if the rest of its family comes too, as in the vitamin's food source (vitamin A with mixed carotenes). "Whole food" supplements are also based on this theory. Scientific studies to solve the mystery of absorbability are inconclusive, but Baby Bistro bets on "au natural!"

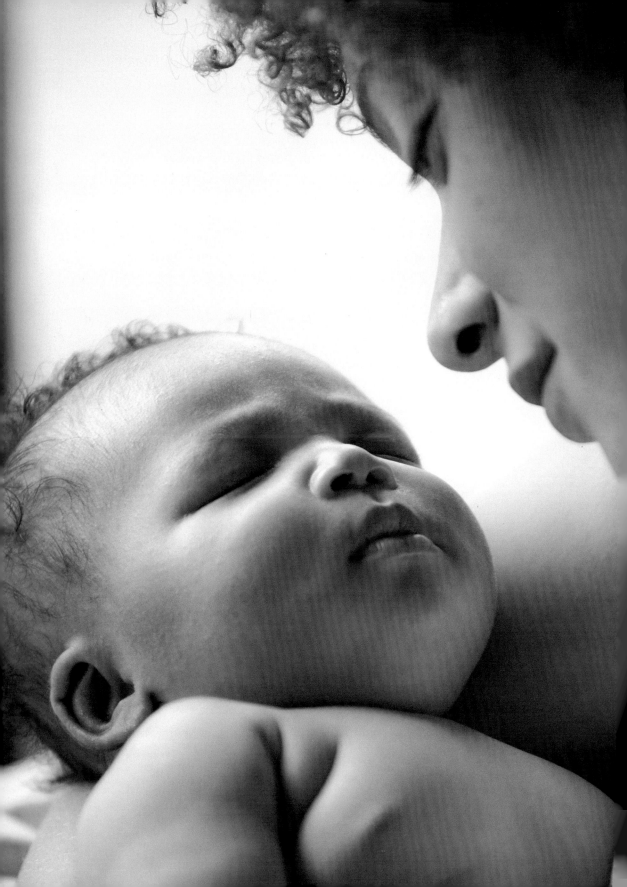

Desserts

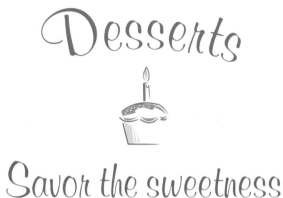

Savor the sweetness

No, you aren't going to find dessert recipes for your baby here. Sweets are something we all love in life, but we don't need to emphasize them in the first year. This final course is the best kind of dessert—calorie-free and more memorable than your all-time favorite sweet. It is a short list of wisdom from generations about how to nurture and hold on to special moments from this incredible first year with your baby.

Just 1 year old
1 short sweet year
And yet to me
You are so dear

Savor the sweetness . . . of this special, fleeting life stage.

- Keep a camera in your diaper bag.
- Trace your baby's hand and foot.
- Record your baby's voice.
- Play classical music.
- Enjoy a nap with your baby.
- Record with video what you don't have time to write about.
- Tape the news or save news clippings from the day your baby was born.

As tired as you are, you will rejoice that you made time for these memories.

The poem below is from an anonymous source and was engraved on my grandmother Lois' first baby spoon, which also serves as our company logo. Sometimes a simple verse is all you need to express a universal emotion.

> *Just one year old*
> *One short sweet year*
> *And yet to me*
> *You are so dear.*

Appendix 1
A Spoonful of Sources

$\mathcal{I}$n addition to stacks of text and scientific research, my home and cyber-libraries include the following list of favorite books and web sites that relate to safe and healthy infant feeding. These resources will be very helpful to answer your specific questions and to broaden your nutrition knowledge.

Appendices

Books

Elbirt, Paula, M.D., *Dr. Paula's Good Nutrition Guide for Babies, Toddlers, and Preschoolers.* Cambridge: Perseus Publishing, 2001.

Joneja, Janice Vickerstaff, PhD, R.D., *Dealing With Food Allergies in Babies and Children.* Boulder, Colo.: Bull Publishing, 2007.

Kleinman, Ronald E., M.D., *Pediatric Nutrition Handbook, 5th Edition.* USA: American Academy of Pediatrics, 2004.

Tamborlane, William V., M.D., *The Yale Guide to Children's Nutrition.* New Haven, Conn.: Yale University Press, 1997.

Vartabedian, Bryan, M.D., F.A.A.P., *First Foods.* New York: St. Martin's, 2001.

Ward, Elizabeth M., M.S., R.D., *Healthy Foods, Healthy Kids.* Avon, Mass.: Adams Media Corporation, 2002.

Web sites

General parenting advice
www.babycenter.com
www.parenting.ivillage.com
www.babyparenting.about.com
www.breastfeeding.com
www.aap.org
www.eatright.org
www.marchofdimes.com

Fish advisories
www.edf.org
www.epa.gov/waterscience/fish

Food allergies
www.foodallergy.org
www.3.niaid.nih.gov
www.celiac.org

Food safety
www.fsis.usda.gov
www.csfsan.fda.gov
www.cspinet.org
My Water's Fluoride:
http://apps.nccd.cdc.gov/MWF/
      Index.asp
www.cdc.gov

Environmental safety
www.niehs.nih.gov/health
www.ewg.org
www.leadtesting.org
www.nrdc.org

Organic foods
www.eatwellguide.org
www.consumersunion.org

Appendix 2
Shopping Simplicity

Many moms tell me they love having a list of suggested brands to help guide them through their choices at the grocery store. If these brands are not available in your area, see the general shopping guidelines in First Course, Shopping Smarts, p. 31.

Appendices

Birth to four months

Infant formulas
Bright Beginnings organic with lipids
Enfamil Lipil with iron
Nestle Good Start natural cultures
bifidus BL
Similac organic DHA and ARA

Four to six months

Baby food section
Earth's Best (organic purées and rice cereal)
Gerber organic whole-grain rice cereal
Healthy Times (organic purées and brown rice cereal)
Organic Baby
Tender Harvest (organic)

Rice section
Bob's Red Mill creamy rice
Erewhon organic brown rice cream
Uncle Ben's ready rice and instant whole-grain brown rice

Frozen food section (for purées)
Birds Eye vegetables
Cascadian Farms organic fruits and vegetables
Sno Pac organic vegetables
Trader Joe's organic fruits and vegetables
Tree of Life organic vegetables
Woodstock Farms organic fruits and vegetables
365 Organic fruits and vegetables

Canned food section (for purées)
Del Monte sliced peaches or pears in 100% juice
Eden organic apple butter
Mott's Whole Kids
Organic low-salt chicken or vegetable broths

Trader Joe's organic, unsweetened applesauce or other organic, unsweetened brands
365 halved apricots in pear juice

Six to eight months

Baby food section
Earth's Best organic barley teething biscuits, multigrain cereal
Gerber organic whole-grain oatmeal, Veggie wagon wheels or puffs
Healthy Times organic maple biscuits for teethers
Teddy Puffs originals, apple cinnamon, mixed-grain cereal
Whole Kids organic raisins

Bread section
Country Hearth white
Earthgrains potato bread
Milbrook white
Milton's healthy gourmet white, potato
Pacific Bakery wheat alternative
Sara Lee (plain mini-bagels, golden potato bread)
Trader Joe's Mom's white, mini-bagels (plain)

Cereal section
Alti Plano organic quinoa
Arrowhead Mills, Nature's Path, Earth's Best, and Whole Kids Organic "O's" brands
Barbara's Bakery Puffins
Bob's Red Mill, millet grits, amaranth
General Mills Cheerios
New Morning Oatios Original
Organic oatmeal brands
Pure & Simple puffed rice
Trader Joe's O's
Rice section
Lundberg organic rice
Trader Joe's brown rice, fully cooked, organic basmati, organic jasmine

Pasta section

Ancient Quinoa Harvest
Bionaturae
Da Vinci Italian Organics
De Bolles corn, rice
DeCecco with spinach
Eden Organic vegetable alphabets
Lundberg rice
Pastariso
TJ's brown rice, organic vegetable
    Radiatore
365 Organic

Cheese section

Borden Double Twist
Cedargrove Family Farm Organic
Frigo Cheese Heads Swirls
Horizon Organic
Kraft Cubes, Twist-Ums
Organic Valley Stringles
Sorrento Stringsters
TJ's sliced yogurt, mild cheddar, jack
Whole Kids organic string cheese
365 Organic cheese slices

Cheese alternatives (may contain casein) section

Galaxy Foods vegan mozzarella, soy,
    American, rice vegan slices
Soy-Station soy cheese
Tofu Rella
Yves Good Slice

Meat section

Freshly sliced deli meats (not
    pre-packaged) or nitrate-free,
    low-sodium packaged deli meat
Lean, ground turkey
Turkey or chicken breasts
Healthy Choice
Wellshire Farms
Diestel Turkey Ranch
Sara Lee

Meat alternatives section

*See also frozen foods for eight to twelve
months. Some brands contain gluten!*
Firm, whole-fat, organic tofu brands
LightLife roast turkey deli
Smart Ground Original
Tofurky Original, roasted
Wildwood tofu veggie burgers, original
Yves veggie turkey deli slices, ground
    round turkey, original

Yogurt section

Organic, whole-fat, plain yogurts
Stir in 100 percent fruit purées!

Nondairy yogurts/milks
Unsweetened, enriched, organic soy
    milk brands (for recipes)
Nancy's soy
Silk Live soy
Stonyfield Farm O'Soy
Wholesoy

Canned food section

Amy's organic light in sodium
Bearitos organic, no salt added
Eden organic (no salt added) beans
Health Valley organic, no salt added
S&W low-salt beans
Trader Joe's reduced sodium

Eight to twelve months

Frozen food section

Alexia julienne sweet potatoes
Amy's organic garden vegetable
    lasagna with rice pasta
Boca meatless patties
Dr. Praeger's CA veggie burgers,
    salmon cakes
Gardenburger Meatless, GardenVegan,
    breakfast sausage
Ian's wheat-free chicken nuggets, fish
    sticks
Lifestream Mesa Sunrise gluten-free
    toaster waffles

Appendices

Morningstar Farms breakfast patties, vegan grillers

Perdue short cuts, carved chicken breast

Trader Joe's turkey pot pie

Tyson oven-roasted diced chicken

Van's all-natural, wheat-free original gourmet waffles

Veggie Medley flame-grilled or original soy burger

Waffle Heaven wheat-free homestyle

Whole Catch salmon burgers

Canned food section

Crown Prince pink salmon or other low-sodium, water-packed, canned wild salmon brands

Mott's Healthy Harvest unsweetened fruit medleys

Santa Cruz organic apple/apricot sauce

Pasta section

Annie's homegrown organic shells and white cheddar, rice pasta and cheddar

Whole Kids organic macaroni and cheese

Snack section

Back to Nature crispy cheddars

Eden Foods brown rice, veggie, or sea vegetable crisps

Edwards organic, unsalted, plain brown rice snaps, vegetable

GenSoy soy crisps, cheddar

Lundberg brown rice organic rice cakes

Natural GH Foods cheddar guppies

Newman's Own Organics wheat and dairy-free fig newtons

Pepperidge Farms boldfish

Robert's American gourmet veggie, smart puffs

Trader Joe's water crackers

Health Valley rice bran

Wasa Oats

365 seaweed rice crackers

Bread section

Food for Life brown rice tortillas, corn tortillas

Nate's organic polenta, original

Rudy's organic spelt tortillas

Tumaro's organic flour tortillas

365 Organic tortillas traditional, corn tortillas

Supplements

Probiotics

Baby's Jarro-Dophilus, Jarrow formulas (Canada)

Nature's Way Primadophilus for children or kids (Springville, Utah)

Nutrition Now Rhino FOS and Acidophilus (Vancouver, Washington)

Ultra Bifidus, DF, Metagenics (San Clemente, California)

Prenatal vitamin/mineral

Duet DHA (prescription prenatal)

OptiNate (prescription prenatal)

NOW prenatal capsules (Bloomingdale, Illinois)

Rainbow Light prenatal, one multivitamin (Santa Cruz, California)

TwinLab prennatal care multivitamin caps (American Fork, Utah)

DHA

Carlson for Kids Very Finest Fish Oil (Arlington Heights, Illinois)

Mead Johnson Expecta LIPIL (Evansville, Indiana)

Nature's Way Neuromins (Springville, Utah)

Source Naturals DHA (Scotts Valley, California)

Appendix 3
A blend of measurements

Liquid ingredients

1 cup = ½ pint = 8 fl oz = 236.5 mL
2 cups = 1 pint = 16 fl oz = 473 mL
4 cups = 1 quart = 32 fl oz = 946 mL
2 pints = 32 fl oz = 1 quart = 0.946 L
4 quarts = 1 gallon = 128 fl oz = 3.784 L

Dry ingredients

3 teaspoons = 1 tablespoon = ½ oz = 14.2g
12 teaspoons = ¾ cup = 6 oz = 170g
2 tablespoons = ⅛ cup = 1 oz = 28.35g
16 tablespoons = 1 cup = 8 oz = ½ lb = 226.8g
4 tablespoons = ¼ cup = 2 oz = 56.7g
32 tablespoons = 2 cups = 16 oz = 1 lb = 453.6g
5 ⅓ tablespoons = ⅓ cup = 2 ¾ oz = 75.6g
64 tablespoons = 4 cups = 32 oz = 2 lbs = 907g
8 tablespoons = ½ cup = 4 oz = 113.4g

Index

Note: Page numbers with an italic t indicate references to a table.

A

Allergies, 76
    and breast-feeding, 12, 39
    checking the labels, 33
    to cheeses, 15
    to chocolate, 15
    common foods that cause,
        10–11
    to eggs, 16
    to fish and shellfish, 18
    and formulas, 44
    to grains, 30
    to nuts, 24
    and prenatal supplements, 117
    symptoms of, 11, 45, 50
    tips for dealing with, 11–12
Arachidonic acid (ARA), 43

B

Baby, weight gain, 48, 62, 84
Bisphenol A (BPA), 27
Bottle-feeding, 14
Breast-feeding
    alcohol and, 38
    breast implants and, 42
    and caffeine, 39
    dieting and, 40
    fats and, 40
    galactagogue, 40
    herbal supplements and, 42
    medications and, 41–42
    nicotine and, 38, 42
Breast milk

    and allergies, 12, 39
    antioxidant levels in, 40
    benefits of, 36–37
    change of taste in, 38
    nutrients in, 39
    and probiotics, 106
    serving suggestions for, 37–38

C

Calories, during pregnancy and
        breast-feeding, 2, 3
Celiac disease, 31
Cereals, 64, 65
    cooking times, 66*t*
    iron-fortified rice, 52
    mixing milk with, 37
    recipes with, 67
    suggested brands of, 126
Cheese, 14–15
    bread, 98
    quesadillas, 96
Combo cuisine, recipes for, 85–94
Constipation, 113, 114

D

Diets
    low carbohydrate, 6
    macrobiotic, 5
    vegan or vegetarian, 5
Docosahexanoic acid (DHA), 43,
        105, 114–115
    suggested brands of, 115, 128

E

Eggs, 16

F

Fats, 4, 48, 63, 84
 and breast-feeding, 40
 low-fat and fat-free products, 20
 partially hydrogenated (trans), 21
Fiber, 3
Finger foods, 64
 with asparagus, 80
 with bananas, 98
 with broccoli, 96
 with butternut squash, 80
 good selections of, 76, 77
 with parsnips, 78, 95
 recipes for, 76–81
 with spinach, 88
 with tofu, 95
Fish, 4, 7
 kinds to avoid, 18
 salmon, 19–20, 98
 tuna, 17
Fluoride, 108–109
Food safety, 7, 51
 choking hazards, 15, 53
 fish advisories, 17
 food storage, 53–54
Formulas
 and docosahexanoic acid
  (DHA), 105
 hypoallergenic, 44
 iron fortified, 45, 107
 lactose-free, 44
 and probiotics, 106
 serving suggestions for, 45
 soy-based, 44
 specialized, 44

 standard cow's milk-based, 43
 suggested brands of, 43, 126
Fruits, 21–22
 high in iron, 116

G

Galactagogue, 40

H

Honey, 22

I

Iron
 deficiency, 107–108
 foods rich in, 63, 116–117
 fortified formulas, 45, 107
 fortified rice-cereal, 52
 sources of, 108

J

Juices, 14

L

Lactation. *See* Breast-feeding;
Breast milk

M

Mashes, 70–71
 with apple, 74–75
 with avocado, 72
 with edamame, 72
 with egg, 72
 recipes for, 72, 74–75
Measurements, conversion, 129
Meats, 22–23

Subject Index

chicken, 88, 90
    cured, 23
    ready-to-eat, 23
    red, 23
    turkey, 80
Milk
    breast (*see* Breast-feeding;
        Breast milk)
    cow's milk, 12–13
    formula (*see* Formulas)
    goat milk, 13
    milk imposters, 13
    soy, 13
Muffins
    with broccoli, 99
    with carrot, 87
    with sweet potato and spinach,
        100

N

Nutrient needs
    from birth to four months, 36*t*
    for eight to twelve months, 84*t*
    for four to six months, 48*t*
    for six to eight months, 62*t*
Nuts, 24

O

Oats and oatmeal
    bars, 96
    biscuits, 77
Organic foods, 24–26

P

Pasta, 78, 90

Pesticides
    foods with high and low
        residues of, 26*t*
    minimizing exposure to, 25–26
Plastics, 27–28
Pregnancy
    caloric intake during, 2, 3
    fiber intake during, 3
    foods to avoid, 6–7
    prenatal supplements (*see*
        Prenatal supplements)
    protein intake during, 2, 3
    recommended weight gain
        during, 2
Prenatal supplements
    and breast-feeding, 37
    ideal amount of vitamins and
        minerals in, 111*t*–112*t*
    shopping for, 117–118
    suggested brands, 114, 128
    suggestions for taking, 113
    vitamin formulations, 118–119
Probiotics, 106–107, 118
    in formulas, 43
    suggested brands, 128
    supplements, 106–107
Proteins
    and allergies, 10
    foods rich in, 3
    gluten, 30–31
    meats, 22–23
    during pregnancy and breast-
        feeding, 2, 3
Purées, 54, 64
    with amaranth, 67
    with apple, 56, 68